Treatment of Affective Disorders in the Elderly

The
PROGRESS IN PSYCHIATRY Series

David Spiegel, M.D., Series Editor

SPRING 1985

The Borderline: Current Empirical Research
Edited by Thomas H. McGlashan, M.D.

Premenstrual Syndrome:
Current Findings and Future Directions
Edited by Howard J. Osofsky, M.D., Ph.D., and Susan J. Blumenthal, M.D.

Treatment of Affective Disorders in the Elderly
Edited by Charles A. Shamoian, M.D., Ph.D.

Treatment of Affective Disorders in the Elderly

Edited by
Charles A. Shamoian, M.D., Ph.D.

American Psychiatric Press, Inc.

1400 K Street, N.W., Suite 505
Washington, DC 20005

Note: The authors have worked to ensure that all information in this book concerning drug dosages, schedules, and routes of administration is accurate as of the time of publication and consistent with standards set by the U.S. Food and Drug Administration and the general medical community. As medical research and practice advance, however, therapeutic standards may change. For this reason and because human and mechanical errors sometimes occur, we recommend that readers follow the advice of a physician who is directly involved in their care or the care of a member of their family.

Manufactured in the United States of America

Library of Congress Cataloging in Publication Data
Main entry under title:

Treatment of affective disorders in the elderly.

(The Progress in psychiatry series)
Based on a symposium held during the 138th Annual Meeting of the American Psychiatric Association in Dallas, Tex., on May 21, 1985.
Includes bibliographies.
1. Affective disorders—Congresses. 2. Affective disorders—Chemotherapy—Congresses. 3. Geriatric psychiatry—Congresses. I. Shamoian, Charles A., 1931– . II. American Psychiatric Association. Meeting (138th : 1985 : Dallas, Tex.) III. Series. [DNLM: 1. Depressive Disorder—drug therapy—congresses. 2. Depressive Disorder—in old age—congresses. WM 171 T7837 1985]
RC537.T736 1985 618.97'68527061 85-6103
ISBN 0-88048-086-6

Contents

Contributors

George S. Alexopoulos, M.D.
Associate Professor of Psychiatry, Cornell University Medical College; and Division of Geriatric Services, New York Hospital–Cornell Medical Center, Westchester Division

John P. Blass, M.D., Ph.D.
Burke Professor of Neurology and Medicine, Department of Neurology, Cornell University Medical College; and Director, Dementia Research Service, Burke Rehabilitation Center

Sylvia Gerson, Ph.D.
Clinical Instructor of Psychiatry, University of South Florida School of Medicine

Robert Greenberg, M.D.
Assistant Professor of Psychiatry, Cornell University Medical College; and Department of Psychiatry, New York Hospital–Cornell Medical Center, Westchester Division

James A. Haycox, M.D.
Department of Psychiatry, McLean Hospital

Lissy F. Jarvik, M.D., Ph.D.
Professor of Psychiatry, University of California Department of Psychiatry and Behavioral Sciences; and Chief, Psychogeriatric Unit, West Los Angeles V.A. Medical Center

Kenneth W. Lieberman, Ph.D.
Department of Pathology, Catholic Medical Center

John R. Lipsey, M.D.
Assistant Professor of Psychiatry, Department of Psychiatry and Behavioral Science and Neuroscience, The Johns Hopkins University School of Medicine

Varda Mei-Tal, M.D.
Brooklyn V.A. Medical Center

Barnett S. Meyers, M.D.
Assistant Professor of Psychiatry, Cornell University Medical College; and Division of Geriatric Services, New York Hospital–Cornell Medical Center, Westchester Division

Thomas R. Price, M.D.
Professor of Neurology, University of Maryland School of Medicine

Robert G. Robinson, M.D.
Department of Psychiatry and Neuroscience, The Johns Hopkins University School of Medicine and University of Maryland

Abdol H. Samiy, M.D.
Professor of Clinical Medicine, Cornell Medical College; and Chief, Division of Medicine, New York Hospital–Cornell Medical Center, Westchester Division

Charles A. Shamoian, M.D., Ph.D.
Professor of Clinical Psychiatry, Cornell Medical College; and Director, Division of Geriatric Services, New York Hospital–Cornell Medical Center, Westchester Division

James E. Spar, M.D.
Assistant Professor of Psychiatry, UCLA School of Medicine

Richard C. Veith, M.D.
Associate Professor, Department of Psychiatry and Behavioral Sciences, University of Washington School of Medicine; and Clinical Investigator, Geriatric Research, Education, and Clinical Center, Seattle V.A. Medical Center

Robert C. Young, M.D.
Assistant Professor of Psychiatry, Cornell University Medical College; and Division of Geriatric Services, New York Hospital–Cornell Medical Center, Westchester Division

Introduction to the Progress in Psychiatry Series

The *Progress in Psychiatry* Series is designed to capture in print the excitement that comes from assembling a diverse group of experts from various locations to examine in detail the newest information about a developing aspect of psychiatry. This series emerged as a collaboration between the American Psychiatric Association's Scientific Program Committee and the American Psychiatric Press, Inc. Great interest was generated by a number of the symposia presented each year at the APA Annual Meeting, and we realized that much of the information presented there, carefully assembled by people who are deeply immersed in a given area, would unfortunately not appear together in print. The symposia sessions at the Annual Meetings provide an unusual opportunity for experts who otherwise might not meet on the same platform to share their diverse viewpoints for a period of three hours. Some new themes are repeatedly reinforced and gain credence, while in other instances disagreements emerge, enabling the audience and now the reader to reach informed decisions about new directions in the field. The *Progress in Psychiatry* Series allows us to publish and capture some of the best of the symposia and thus provide an in-depth treatment of specific areas which might not otherwise be presented in broader review formats.

The symposia are selected on the basis of review by the Symposium Subcommittee of the Scientific Program Committee. From the approximately 80 symposia a year selected for presentation at the Annual Meeting, we choose approximately 10 percent which are deemed to be of especially high quality and to have interest to readers as well as meeting participants. After review by the American Psychiatric Press, we invite the authors to submit their papers as manuscripts for publication. We make every effort to expedite the publishing process so that books in the *Progress in Psychiatry* Series will be available as close as possible to the time of presentation at the Annual Meeting.

We believe the *Progress in Psychiatry* Series will provide you with an opportunity to review timely new information in specific fields of interest as they are developing. We hope you find that the excitement of the presentations is captured in the written word and that this book proves to be informative and enjoyable reading.

David Spiegel, M.D.
Series Editor
Progress in Psychiatry Series

Introduction

Depression in the elderly is probably underdiagnosed and frequently misdiagnosed. The true incidence and prevalence of this affective disorder in the elderly is still equivocal. The figures reported vary from report to report depending upon the site of the study and the source of the patients (inpatient, outpatient clinic, or community) (Blazer and Williams 1980; Gurland et al. 1980). The diagnosis of depression in the elderly is often complicated by the presence of concomitant medical and neurological illnesses. At age 65, patients usually have one chronic medical problem, and at age 75 the elderly suffer from at least two. The medical illnesses can present as depression, induce or aggravate a preexisting affective disorder, or mask the underlying depressive state. To complicate the clinical picture, some appropriately prescribed medications may augment the depression. These medications include, to mention only a few, reserpine, propranolol, alpha methyl dopa, L-dopa, and indomethacin (Hirschfeld and Klerman 1979). At any point in time, the elderly patient is ingesting seven to 10 different prescribed medications not including over-the-counter preparations or alcohol.

Regardless of the clinical presentation or chief complaint, all elderly patients should be assessed for depression, which not infrequently presents in the absence of a dysphoric mood. Depression is associated with an increased morbidity and successful suicide. Although the elderly presently account for only 12 percent of the general population in the United States, they are responsible for 25 percent of annually completed suicides (Blazer 1982). Unfortunately depression in the elderly is often perceived by both the patient and family as a normal component of old age. To be noted is that even though this phase of the life cycle is fraught with all sorts of losses, not all elderly experience the pathological state of depression. However, for those who do suffer from this illness, there is hope. With the increase in scientific knowledge of the biology and treatment of depression, a very high percentage of those so afflicted can now be effectively and safely treated.

This book presents some of the current approaches to the biology, diagnosis, and treatment of depression in the elderly, frequently complicated by the presence of concomitant medical problems. With the exception of that on kidney and lithium therapy in the elderly, these chapters were originally presented as part of a symposium on "The Treatment of Affective Disorders in the Elderly" at the Annual Meeting of the American Psychiatric Association, held in Dallas, Texas, in May 1985.

The first chapter, "Biological Studies in Depression with Reversible Dementia," by Alexopoulos et al., highlights the complex relationship of depression and dementia. Platelet monoamine oxidase (MAO) activity and the dexamethasone suppression test (DST) have been studied to achieve some understanding of the pathophysiology of depression with reversible dementia. Based on the MAO studies the authors conclude that "at least in some elderly patients, a reversible dementia syndrome develops when pathophysiological changes of depression are added to an asymptomatic biologic process associated with degenerative dementia." Unfortunately the DST, as in other reported studies, was found to be of practically no use in clarifying the diagnostic differential dilemma of depression and dementia.

The second chapter, "Delusional Depression in the Elderly," by Meyers et al., deals with many of the important clinical issues so frequently encountered in the treatment of elderly patients with delusional depression. Up to this point in time, the issue of delusional depression in the elderly had not been investigated. These authors, in their naturalistic study, highlight the frequency of this phenomenon in the elderly and reinforce the efficacy of electroconvulsive treatment of delusional depression.

The third chapter, "Outcome of Drug Treatment in Depressed Patients Over the Age of Fifty," by Jarvik and Gerson, reviews in depth the currently available studies. To quote these investigators, "It seems paradoxical that, despite the high frequency of depression among them, persons over the age of 65 years have been excluded from treatment-outcome research." Even though as clinicians we use antidepressants daily, the authors state, "Data on treatment outcome need to be gathered on patients specified by age, classified with diagnostic vigor, etc." This review certainly emphasizes the need for additional studies in geriatric depression and specifically the need for scientific longitudinal studies in treated depressives.

The next two chapters, by Veith and Spar, deal with the effect of antidepressants on the cardiovascular system and the use of these drugs (including stimulants, lithium, monoamine oxidase inhibitors, and the newer antidepressants) in patients with cardiovascular disease. These authors clearly and systematically review the current literature based on the topic. Guidelines for the clinician are provided. Both authors conclude that although these drugs are not without unwanted side effects, they can be used effectively in patients with cardiovascular problems, with careful and proper monitoring.

The sixth chapter, by Robinson et al., deals with the studies conducted by this group on mood disorders in post-stroke patients. Based on animal and clinical studies the conclusion is drawn that "left frontal lesions are strongly related to depression and the closer the lesion is to the frontal pole the more severe the depression." Moreover, the clinical studies have clearly shown that these depressions are treatable with the tricyclic antidepressant nortriptyline.

The final chapter, "Kidney and Lithium Therapy in the Elderly" by Samiy, reviews a very important and controversial issue—the effect of lithium on the kidney in the elderly. Lithium is used very frequently in affective disorders in both young and old patients. However, very little emphasis has been placed on the use of lithium in the ill aged. This chapter provides the physician with clinical guidelines for monitoring kidney functions in the elderly, who are not uncommonly on salt-restricted diets or diuretics.

This book should provide the reader with a better understanding of the multifaceted problems with which he or she will be confronted in treating the elderly depressive. The controversial issues of biological markers, diagnosis, treatment, and treatment outcome in depression in the elderly, often complicated by medical illnesses, are highlighted. It is to be hoped that this book will stimulate the reader to pursue additional studies in this area and will provide a scientific, rational basis for the treatment of depression in the elderly, which so often challenges our diagnostic skills and clinical acumen.

Charles A. Shamoian, M.D., Ph.D.

REFERENCES

Blazer DG, Williams CD: The epidemiology of dysphoria and depression in an elderly population. Am J Psychiatry 137:439–444, 1980

Blazer DG: Depression in Late Life. St. Louis, C.V. Mosby Co., 1982

Gurland B, Dean L, Cross P, et al.: The epidemiology of depression and dementia in the elderly: the use of multiple indicators of these conditions, in Psychopathology in the Aged. Edited by Cole JB, Barrett JE. New York, Raven Press, 1980, pp 37–60

Hirschfeld RMA, Klerman G: Treatment of depression in the elderly. Geriatrics 34:51–57, 1979

Chapter 1

Biological Studies in Depression with Reversible Dementia

George S. Alexopoulos, M.D.
Robert C. Young, M.D.
James A. Haycox, M.D.
John P. Blass, M.D., Ph.D.
Kenneth W. Lieberman, Ph.D.
Charles A. Shamoian, M.D., Ph.D.

Chapter 1

Biological Studies in Depression with Reversible Dementia

Depression and dementia are common in the elderly. Dementia occurs in up to 20 percent of the elderly population (Gurland et al. 1980) and its most common cause is Alzheimer's disease (Schneck et al. 1982). The prevalence of severe depression in elderly people living in the community is 2.5 to 3.7 percent, while milder depressive syndromes occur in 4.5 to 13 percent of the aged population (Blazer and Williams 1980; Gurland et al. 1980).

Early literature has suggested that some patients with irreversible dementia may develop depressive syndrome (Roth 1955). At least three studies of demented patients diagnosed through brain autopsy or biopsy indicate that a subpopulation among them had depression (Sim and Sussman 1965; Coblentz et al. 1973; Rosen et al. 1979). Rosen et al. (1979) have observed that depressive symptomatology develops in Alzheimer's disease patients with autopsy-confirmed diagnosis, and challenged the notion that depression occurs primarily in multi-infarct dementia (Hachinski et al. 1975). Elderly patients with organic brain syndrome have been shown to have more depressive symptomatology than same-age cognitively intact patients (Miller 1980). In a study of demented nursing-home residents, 25 percent had severe and 56 percent mild depressive symptomatology (Ernst et al. 1977), while in another study (Reifler et al. 1982), of demented patients attending a geriatric clinic, 23 percent met Research Diagnostic Criteria for major depressive disorder (Spitzer et al. 1977).

Cognitive dysfunction of varying degree occurs in depression

This work has been supported by funds of the Department of Psychiatry, Cornell University Medical College and the Westchester Division of the New York Hospital and by funds from the Xerox Foundation.

We thank L. Waldhorn, M.A., and L. Rowan, R.N., C.N.P. for their assistance in the collection of data.

(Friedman 1964; Kiloh 1961; Post 1975). Mild dysfunction may be expressed as subjective difficulty in thinking and a mild decline in performance scores on the Wechsler's Adult Intelligence Scale (Ford 1975). Severe cognitive dysfunction with disturbance of recent memory, disorientation, loss of concentration, and poor knowledge of current events has also been described in depressed patients (Kiloh 1961; Post 1975; Folstein and McHugh 1978; Wells 1979; Rabins et al. 1984). This picture is often difficult to distinguish from irreversible dementia but it subsides when symptoms of depression remit (Kiloh 1961; Folstein and McHugh 1978). The relationship between dementia and depression raises the question whether common or synergistic brain abnormalities contribute in the pathophysiology of these two disorders.

Peripheral measures of brain function have been used to investigate affective disorders and primary degenerative dementia. Platelet monoamine oxidase (MAO) is an enzyme that catabolizes biogenic amines and participates in the intraneuronal regulation of these substances in the brain (Kopin 1964; Spector et al. 1967). Platelet MAO activity has been used as an index of central monoaminergic activity in the investigation of psychiatric disorders (Sandler et al. 1981; Fowler et al. 1982). Most studies indicate that patients with a bipolar affective disorder have increased platelet MAO activity compared to normal controls (Sandler et al. 1981; Fowler et al. 1982), while contradictory findings have been reported in unipolar depression (Marbach et al. 1981). Recently, it has been shown that elderly depressed women, with onset of illness before the senium, may have lower platelet MAO activity than same-age depressives with late onset of illness or normal control subjects (Alexopoulos et al. 1984a). Elevation in MAO activity has been found in both the platelets (Adolfsson et al. 1980; Alexopoulos et al. 1984b) and the brain of patients with primary degenerative dementia (Adolfsson et al. 1980). A weak but significant correlation has been reported between platelet MAO activity and depressive symptomatology in patients with primary degenerative dementia (Alexopoulos et al. 1984c). There are no studies, to our knowledge, of platelet MAO activity in depressed patients with a reversible dementia syndrome.

Hyperactivity of the hypothalamic/pituitary/adrenal axis (HPA) has been reported in depression (Carroll et al. 1981; Coppen et al. 1983). The dexamethasone suppression test (DST) has been found abnormal in a considerable percentage of depressives and reflects hyperactivity of the HPA axis in this disorder (Carroll 1981; Coppen et al. 1983). Elderly depressed patients have an abnormal DST more frequently than younger depressives (Alexopoulos et al. 1984d). It has been suggested that the DST may be useful in the diagnosis of depression with reversible dementia (Rudorfer and Clayton 1982; McAllister 1982; Jenike 1983). Recently, abnormal DSTs have been reported in a considerable number of elderly demented patients (Raskind et al. 1982; Spar and Gerner 1982; Balldin et al. 1983; Carnes et al. 1983; Coppen et al. 1983; Katonah and Aldridge, personal communication; Keith 1984), but there has been no systematic effort to study DST in depressed patients with reversible dementia.

Platelet MAO activity has been measured and the DST has been administered in a large population of elderly psychiatric patients in order to elucidate the pathophysiology of depression with reversible dementia. An additional goal has been to determine whether the DST can distinguish patients with depression and dementia who improve cognitively when their affective symptoms improve from those who remain demented.

METHOD

The patient subjects were geriatric psychiatric patients with major depression and primary degenerative dementia. Diagnosis was made by two research psychiatrists using the *Diagnostic and Statistical Manual of Mental Disorders, Third Edition* (DSM-III). Depression was further subclassified according to Research Diagnostic Criteria (RDC) (Spitzer et al. 1978). The 24-item Hamilton Depression Rating Scale (HDRS) (Hamilton 1960) was used to rate depressive symptomatology, and the Cognitive Capacity Screening Examination (CCSE) (Jacobs et al. 1977) was used to quantify cognitive dysfunction. Family history of psychiatric disorders was classified according to Family History-Research Diagnostic Criteria (FH-RDC) (Spitzer and Endicott 1976); based on information obtained from patients and family members.

Subjects receiving insulin, nitroglycerine, guanethidine, L-dopa, epinephrine, amphetamine, lithium, neuroleptics, tricyclic antidepressants, and MAO inhibitors were excluded from the MAO studies because these drugs have been reported to influence platelet MAO activity (Robinson and Nies 1980). Subjects on reserpine, spironolactone, anticonvulsants, and barbiturates were excluded from the DST study because these agents may lead to a falsely positive DST (Carroll et al. 1981).

Clinical and laboratory staff were blind to each others' data. For the platelet MAO assay, blood samples were collected between 8:00 and 10:00 A.M. and coded. Duplicate platelet pellets were prepared by a series of centrifugations. A modified version of the assay used by Bockar et al. (1974) was employed. According to this method, platelet MAO activity is estimated by determining the amount of ^{14}C radioactive benzylamine metabolized by the platelet MAO. Protein concentration was measured by the Lowry method (1951). The platelet MAO activity is expressed in nanomoles per hour per milligram of protein.

For the DST, dexamethasone (1 mg) was administered orally at 11:00 P.M. Blood (5 ml) was obtained at 4:00 P.M. on the following day for the determination of plasma cortisol. Samples were centrifuged immediately and frozen at −20°C. Plasma cortisol was determined within one week from sampling time using a radioimmunoassay (Stokes et al. 1984).

All subjects were followed and rated periodically with the HDRS and the CCSE. Subjects with major depression and dementia whose cognitive dysfunction improved (ΔCCSE > 3, final CCSE > 23) when symptoms of depression subsided (ΔHDRS > 10, final HDRS < 12) were classified as depression with reversible dementia (DRD). Subjects who met criteria for major depression and primary degenerative dementia and had a persistent cognitive dysfunction (CCSE < 24) even after improvement of depressive symptomatology (ΔHDRS > 10, final HDRS < 12) were considered to have both disorders (DD).

Statistical analysis of continuous data was performed using the Student's *t*-test and one-way analysis of variance (ANOVA). Post hoc comparison of means was done with the Neuman–Keuls method. Categorical data were analyzed, using the chi-square test with Yates' correction. The reported significance levels are two-tailed.

RESULTS

Platelet MAO Activity Study

Subjects participating in this study were all geriatric depressed inpatients who had been off psychotropic drugs for at least 10 days. None of the subjects had history of migraine, diabetes, cirrhosis, malignancies, epilepsy, Huntington's chorea, or history and blood values suggestive of pyridoxine or iron deficiency, which influence platelet MAO activity (Robinson and Nies 1980; Fowler et al. 1982). Platelet counts were within normal limits.

Platelet MAO activity was assayed in 47 cognitively intact patients (CCSE > 23) with major depression, 23 patients with DRD, and 14 patients with DD. Severity of depression was comparable in the three groups, who had mean + SD pretreatment HDRS scores of 29.4 + 7.1, 32.7 + 7.6, and 33.1 + 8.0, respectively. Cognitively intact depressed patients had a mean + SD pretreatment CCSE score of 27.1 + 1.9, while the mean pretreatment CCSE scores of DRD and DD patients were 19.7 + 3.0 and 16.6 + 5.2.

Platelet MAO activity was significantly different in nondemented elderly subjects with major depression, DRD subjects, and DD subjects (Table 1). Post hoc comparison of means showed that DRD and DD patients had significantly higher platelet MAO activity than cognitively intact depressives ($p < 0.05$). This difference could not be attributed to different age of subjects in the three groups.

In the combined group of depressed patients, platelet MAO activity was similarly distributed among the RDC depression subtypes (psychotic, endogenous, agitated, retarded, situational, incapacitated, recurrent) ($F = 0.61$, $df = 6, 331$, $p > 0.05$). The range of mean platelet MAO activity (nanomoles of ^{14}C-benzylamine per hour per milligram of protein) among the RDC subtypes of depressives without cognitive impairment was 44.5 to 52.6, DRD 61.6 to 71.8, and DD 73.5 to 84.7. Therefore differences in platelet MAO activity between depressives without cognitive impairment, DRD, and DD subjects cannot be attributed to differences in affective symptomatology of this sample.

Platelet MAO activity is reported to be higher in women than in men (Robinson and Nies 1980). To control for the influence of sex, the values of women were compared separately. A significant difference was found between platelet MAO activity (nanomoles of ^{14}C benzylamine per hour per milligram of protein) of elderly depressed women without dementia ($N = 37$), DRD ($N = 20$), and DD

Table 1. Platelet MAO Activity on Elderly Hospitalized Patients with Major Depression

Group	Age (years)	Platelet MAO Activity (nmol/hour/mg protein)
Depression without dementia ($N = 47$)	72.0 ± 8.0	50.3 ± 20.2*
Depression with reversible dementia (DRD) ($N = 23$)	74.7 ± 5.5	69.3 ± 23.8
Depression and primary degenerative dementia (DD) ($N = 14$)	74.2 ± 6.3	80.5 ± 17.5

Note. Data are means ± SD.
*One-way ANOVA: $F = 14.05$, $df = 2, 81$, $p < 0.001$.

female subjects ($N = 14$). ($F = 11.47$, $df = 2.68$, $p < 0.001$). Post hoc comparison of means showed that platelet MAO activity was similar in women with DRD (mean: 69.0, SD: 24.1) and DD (mean: 78.6, SD: 16.7). These values were significantly higher than those of cognitively intact depressed women (mean: 50.8, SD: 20.9). All female subjects were postmenopausal; therefore, platelet MAO activity was not influenced by the hormonal changes that take place during the menstrual cycle (Robinson and Nies 1980). There were not enough male subjects for similar comparisons.

DST Study

DST was performed in 43 patients with major depression who had no cognitive dysfunction (CCSE > 23), 41 patients with primary degenerative dementia without substantial depressive symptomatology (HDRS < 12), and in 42 patients who met criteria for both major depression and dementia. All subjects were within 20 percent of their ideal body weights.

Elderly patients with major depression without cognitive dysfunction (67.4 percent) had abnormal DSTs more frequently than nondepressed patients with primary degenerative dementia (34.1 percent) ($x_c = 8.03$, $df = 1$, $p < 0.001$). In the group of depressives, dexamethasone suppressors and dexamethasone nonsuppressors had similar depressive symptomatology (HDRS mean: 27.4, SD: 10.4 versus mean: 27.2, SD: 7.4) and cognitive performance (CCSE mean: 27.9, SD: 1.8 versus mean: 27.9, SD: 0.3) symptamatology prior to treatment. Patients with primary degenerative dementia who suppressed normally had comparable depressive (HDRS mean: 7.1, SD: 7.6) and cognitive ratings (CCSE mean: 7.3, SD: 7.1) with demented dexamethasone nonsuppressors (HDRS mean: 9.6, SD: 6.8 and CCSE mean: 9.8, SD: 6.8).

Elderly patients who met criteria for both depression and dementia ($N = 42$) had abnormal DST more frequently (73.8 percent) than patients with primary degenerative dementia without depression ($x_c = 11.60$, $df = 1$, $p < 0.001$). After antidepressant treatment 26 patients met criteria for DRD and 16 were classified as DD. DRD subjects had higher CCSE scores before treatment (mean: 19.4, SD: 3.0) than DD subjects (CCSE mean: 15.7 SD: 4.6), ($t = 3.07$, $df = 35$, $p < 0.005$). Severity of depression prior to treatment was similar in DRD and DD subjects (HDRS mean: 30.9, SD: 8.0 versus mean: 30.7, SD: 7.0). The frequency of abnormal DST was comparable in DRD (76.9 percent) and DD (68.7 percent) female subjects ($x_c = 0.05$, $df = 1$, $p > 0.05$). In the DRD group cognitive dysfunction was similarly distributed between dexamethasone suppressors and nonsuppressors; there was, however, a trend toward higher HDRS scores in dexamethasone nonsuppressors compared to suppressors ($t = 2.04$, $df = 24$, $p < 0.1$) (Table 2).

DISCUSSION

In this sample, elderly depressed patients with reversible dementia had a cognitive dysfunction similar to that reported by others (Folstein and McHugh 1978; Rabins et al. 1984). Platelet MAO activity in depressed patients with reversible dementia was as high in patients with depression and primary degenerative dementia. The values of both these groups are comparable with platelet MAO activity of a sample of patients with primary degenerative dementia from the same hospital reported elsewhere (Alexopoulos et al. 1984c).

Approximately one-third of patients with primary degenerative dementia had abnormal DSTs. This is somewhat lower than the percentage reported by others (Raskind et al. 1982; Spar and Gerner 1982; Balldin et al. 1983; Carnes et al. 1983; Coppen et al. 1983; Katona and Aldridge, 1984; Keith 1984). A higher percentage of

Table 2. Clinical Ratings of Elderly Patients with Major Depression and Cognitive Dysfunction

Group	DST Suppressors	DST Nonsuppressors
Major depression and dementia ($N = 42$)		
HDRS*	26.2 ± 6.0	32.5 ± 7.3
CCSE†	16.5 ± 4.4	18.5 ± 3.9
Depression with reversible dementia (DRD) ($N = 26$)		
HDRS	25.5 ± 5.6	32.6 ± 7.9
CCSE	17.7 ± 4.5	19.9 ± 2.4
Major depression and primary degenerative dementia (DD) ($N = 16$)		
HDRS	27.0 ± 7.1	30.5 ± 7.2
CCSE	15.2 ± 4.3	16.0 ± 4.9

Note. Data are means ± SD.
*24-item Hamilton Depression Rating Scale.
†Cognitive Capacity Screening Examination.

abnormal DST may have been obtained if more postdexamethasone plasma cortisol samples were obtained.

The presence of abnormal DST in primary degenerative dementia and depression suggests that common abnormalities exist in subgroups of patients suffering from these disorders. Autopsy studies indicate that patients with primary degenerative dementia have reduced norepinephrine levels in several brain areas (Adolfsson et al. 1979; Carlsson et al. 1979; Bondareff et al. 1982), while less direct clinical studies suggest a dysfunction in brain norepinephrine neurotransmission in some depressives (Zis and Goodwin 1982). Norepinephrine participates in the regulation of the HPA axis by tonically inhibiting the corticotropin releasing factor (Reichlin 1981). Therefore, reduced norepinephrine in the hypothalamus may result in abnormal DST. It is likely that reduction of norepinephrine is the common dysfunction resulting in abnormal DST in depression and in primary degenerative dementia. This suggestion is in line with our previously reported finding that depression interacts with aging to increase the frequency of DST nonsuppression, since reduced brain norepinephrine concentration has been reported in both conditions. Further studies, however, are needed in order to clarify the relationship of norepinephrine to abnormal DST in these disorders of the elderly.

Aging leads to an increase of platelet and brain MAO activity (Robinson and Nies 1980) and a decrease in several brain neurotransmitters including norepinephrine (Carlsson et al. 1979). Platelet and brain MAO activity are even more elevated and brain norepinephrine levels are further decreased in patients with primary degenerative dementia (Adolfsson et al. 1979; Carlsson et al. 1979; Adolfsson et al. 1980; Alexopoulos et al. 1984b). Based on the observation that the elderly are more prone to developing depression with reversible dementia (Post 1975; Folstein and McHugh 1978; Rabins et al. 1984), a possible speculation is that normal aged individuals with extreme changes in MAO and brain norepinephrine values are predisposed to developing a transient dementia syndrome when they become depressed. It also may be likely that some patients with reversible dementia have increased platelet MAO activity in association with an underlying primary degenerative dementia disease process and that the dementia becomes evident when the pathophysiological changes of depression are added. Follow-up studies are needed to show whether depressed patients with reversible dementia and high platelet MAO activity have a higher probability of developing primary degenerative dementia.

Neither platelet MAO activity nor DST appear helpful in the differential diagnosis of patients with depression and dementia. In most cases, clinicians are able to distinguish this condition from depression without dementia and from dementia without significant depression. What is sometimes problematic is to identify those patients with depression and dementia who will have cognitive improvement when their depression is brought to remission. Since platelet MAO activity and DST cannot predict the outcome of dementia in depressed patients with cognitive dysfunction, their clinical usefulness is limited.

SUMMARY

The relationship between depression and dementia is complex. Depression occurs frequently in patients with dementia and conversely, some elderly depressed patients may develop a severe but reversible cognitive dysfunction. We studied platelet monoamine oxidase (MAO) and the 1-mg dexamethasone suppression test (DST) in an effort to elucidate the pathophysiology of depression with reversible dementia.

Platelet MAO activity has been used as an index of brain monoaminergic activity. Patients with major depression and a reversible dementia syndrome (DRD) (N = 23) had platelet MAO activity similar to that of depressives who also had primary degenerative dementia (PDD) (N = 14). However, both these groups had significantly higher platelet MAO activity than major depressives without cognitive impairment (N = 47) ($p < .001$). This finding is consistent with the idea that, at least in some elderly patients, a reversible dementia syndrome develops when pathophysiological changes of depression are added to an asymptomatic biologic process associated with degenerative dementia.

Abnormal DST has been found in depression and reflects a disinhibition of the hypothalamic/pituitary/adrenal axis (HPA). In our studies, patients with PDD (N = 41) had abnormal DST less frequently (34.1 percent) than elderly patients with major depression without cognitive dysfunction (N = 43, 67.4 percent) ($p < .001$). However, a similar percentage of abnormal DST was found in DRD (N = 26, 76.9 percent) and in depressed patients who remained demented even after improvement of depressive symptoms (N = 16, 68.7 percent). This suggests that common brain abnormalities exist in these two disorders. Abnormal DST may be of little help to clinicians in the differential diagnosis of elderly patients with depression and dementia.

REFERENCES

Adolfsson R, Gottfries CG, Roos BE, et al: Changes in the brain catecholamines in patients with dementia of Alzheimer's type. Br J Psychiatry 135:216–223, 1979

Adolfsson R, Gottfries CG, Oreland L, et al: Increased activity of brain and platelet monoamine oxidase in dementia of Alzheimer's type. Life Sci 27:1029–1034, 1980

Alexopoulos GS, Lieberman KW, Young RC, et al: Platelet monoamine oxidase in geriatric depressed women. Am J Psychiatry 140:1276–1278, 1984a

Alexopoulos GS, Lieberman KW, Young RC: Platelet MAO activity in primary degenerative dementia. Am J. Psychiatry 141:97–99, 1984b

Alexopoulos GS, Lieberman KW, Young RC, et al: Monoamines and monoamine oxidase in primary degenerative dementia, in Dementia in the Elderly. Edited by Shamoian CA, Washington, DC, American Psychiatric Press, 1984c.

Alexopoulos GS, Young RC, Kocsis JH, et al: Dexamethasone suppression test in geriatric depression. Biol Psychiatry, 19:783–787, 1984d.

Balldin J, Gottfries CG, Karlsson I, Dexamethasone suppression test and serum prolactin in dementia disorders. Br J Psychiatry 142:277–281, 1983

Blazer D, Williams CD: Epidemiology of dysphoria and depression in an elderly population. Am J. Psychiatry 137:439–444, 1980

Bockar J, Roth R, Heninger G: Increased human platelet monoamine oxidase during lithium carbonate therapy. Life Sci 15:2109–2118, 1974

Bondareff W, Montjoy CQ, Roth M: Loss of neurons of origin of the adrenergic projection to cerebral cortex (nucleus locus cerulens) in senile dementia. Neurology 32:164–168, 1982

Carlsson A, Adolfsson R, Aquilonius SM, et al: Biogenic amines in human brain in normal aging, senile dementia and chronic alcoholism, in Ergot Compounds and Brain Function: Neuroendocrine and Neuropsychiatric Aspects. Edited by Goldstein M. New York, Raven Press, 1979

Carnes M, Smith JC, Kalin NH, et al: The dexamethasone suppression test in demented outpatients with and without depression. Psychiatry Res 9: 337–344, 1983

Carroll MS, Feinberg M, Greden JF, et al: A specific laboratory test for the diagnosis of melancholia: standardization, validation and clinical utility. Arch Gen Psychiatry 38:15–22, 1981

Coblentz JM, Mattis S, Zingesser Kasoff SS, et al: Presenile dementia. Arch Neurol 29:299–308, 1973

Coppen A, Abou-Saleh M, Milne P, et al: Dexamethasone suppression test in depression and other pscyhiatric illness. Br J Psychiatry 142:498–504, 1983

Ernst P, Badash D, Beran B, et al: Incidence of mental illness in the aged: unmasking the effects of diagnosis of chronic brain syndrome. J Am Geriatr Soc 8:371–375, 1977

Folstein MF, McHugh PM: Dementia syndrome of depression, in Alzheimer's Disease: Senile Dementia and Related Disorders (Aging, vol 7). Edited by Katzman R, Terry RD, Bick KL. New York, Raven Press, 1978, pp. 87–93

Ford H: Involutional melancholia, in Comprehensive Textbook of Psychiatry III, 2nd ed. Edited by Friedman AM, Kaplan HI, Sadock BJ. Baltimore, Williams & Wilkins, 1975, pp 1030–1032

Fowler CJ, Tipton KF, MacKay AVP, et al: Human platelet monoamine oxidase—a useful enzyme in the study of psychiatric disorders? Neuroscience 7:1577–1594, 1982

Friedman AS: Minimal effects of severe depression on cognitive functioning. Abnormal Social Psychology 69:237–243, 1964

Gurland B, Dean L, Cross P, et al: The epidemiology of depression and dementia in the elderly: the use of multiple indicators of these conditions, in Psychotherapy in the Aged. Edited by Cole JO, Barrett JE. New York, Raven Press, 1980

Hachinski VC, Iliff LD, Zilkha E, et al: Cerebral blood flow in dementia. Arch Neurol 32:632–637, 1975

Hamilton M: A rating scale for depression. J. Neurol Neurosurg Psychiatry 23:56–62, 1960

Jacobs JW, Bernhardt MR, Delgado A, et al: Screening for organic mental syndromes in the medically ill. Ann Intern Med 86:40–46, 1977

Jenike MA: Dexamethasone suppression test as a clinical aid in elderly depressed patients. J Am Geriatr Soc 31:45–48, 1983

Katona CL, Aldridge CR: Dexamethasone suppression test and dementia (letter). Br J Psychiatry 144:333, March 1984

Keith IG: Clinical use of the DST in a psychogeriatric population. Br J Psychiatry 145:389–393, 1984

Kiloh LG: Pseudodementia. Acta Psychiatr Scand 3:336–351, 1961

Kopin J: Storage and metabolism of catecholamines: the role of monoamine oxidase. Pharmacol Rev 16:179–191, 1964

Lowry OH, Rosebrough, NH, Farr AL, et al: Protein measurement with the folin phenol reagent. J Biol Chem 193:265–275, 1951

McAllister TW, Ferrell RB, Price TRP, et al: The dexamethasone suppression test in two patients with severe depressive pseudo-dementia. Am J Psychiatry 139:479–481, 1982

Marbach M, Diebold K, Friedl W, et al: Platelet MAO activity in patients with affective psychosis and their first-degree relatives. Pharmacopsychiatria 14:87–93, 1981

Miller NE: The measurement of mood in senile brain disease: examiner ratings and self-reports, in Psychopathology of the Aged. Edited by Cole JO, Barrett JE. New York, Raven Press, 1980, pp 97–118

Post F: Diagnosis of depression in geriatric patients and treatment modalities appropriate for the population, in Depression: Behavioral, Biochemical, Diagnosis, and Treatment Concepts. Edited by Gallant DM, Simpson GM. New York, Spectrum Publications, 1975

Rabins PV, Merchant A, Nedstadt G: Criteria for diagnosing reversible dementia caused by depression: validation by a 2-year following. Br J Psychiatry 144:488–492, 1984

Raskind M, Peskind E, Rivard MF, et al: Dexamethasone suppression test and cortisol circadian rhythm in primary degenerative dementia. Am J Psychiatry 139:1468–1471, 1982

Reichlin S: Neuroendocrinology, in Textbook of Endocrinology, 6th edition. Edited by Williams RH. Philadelphia, W. B. Saunders, 1981, pp 419–589

Reifler BV, Larson E, Hanley R: Coexistence of cognitive impairment and depression in geriatric outpatients. Am J Psychiatry 139:623–626, 1982

Robinson DS, Nies A: Demographic, biologic and other variables affecting monoamine oxidase activity. Schizophr Bull 6:298–307, 1980

Rosen WG, Terry RD, Fuld PA, et al: Pathological verification of ischemic score in differentation of dementias. Ann Neurol 7:486–488, 1979

Roth M: The natural history of mental disorder in old age. Journal of Mental Science 101:281–301, 1955

Rudorfer MV, Clayton PJ: Pseudodementia: use of the DST in diagnosis and treatment monitoring. Psychosomatics 23:429–431, 1982

Sandler M, Reveley MA, Glover V: Human platelet monoamine oxidase activity in health and disease: a review. J Clin Pathol 34:292–302, 1981

Schneck MK, Reisberg R, Ferris SH: An overview of current concepts of Alzheimer's disease. Am J Psychiatry 139:165–173, 1982

Sim M, Sussman I: Alzheimer's disease: its natural history and differential diagnosis. J Nerv Ment Dis 135:489–499, 1965

Spar JE, Gerner R: Does the dexamethasone suppression test distinguish dementia from depression? Am J Psychiatry 139:238–240, 1982

Spector S, Gordon R, Sjoerdsma A, et al: End product inhibition of tyrosine hydroxylase as a possible mechanism for regulation of norepinephrine synthesis. Mol Pharmacol 3:549–555, 1967

Spitzer R, Endicott J: Family History Research—Diagnostic Criteria. New York, Biometrics Research Division of New York State Psychiatric Institute, 1976

Spitzer R, Endicott J, Robins E: Research Diagnostic Criteria for Selected Psychiatric Disorders, 3rd ed. New York, Biometrics Research Division of New York State Psychiatric Institute, 1977

Stokes PE, Stoll PM, Koslow SH, et al: Pretreatment DST and hypothalamic–pituitary–adrenocortical function in depressed patients and comparison groups. A multicenter study. Arch Gen Psychiatry 41:257–267, 1984

Wells CE: Pseudodementia. Am J Psychiatry 136:895–900, 1979

Zis AP, Goodwin FK: The amine hypothesis, in Handbook of Affective Disorders. Edited by Paykel ES. New York, Guilford Press, 1982

Chapter 2

Delusional Depression in the Elderly

Barnett S. Meyers, M.D.
Robert Greenberg, M.D.
Varda Mei-Tal, M.D.

Chapter 2

Delusional Depression in the Elderly

Studies of the relationship of delusions to major depressive episodes have failed to identify age as a factor contributing to this association. Delusional and nondelusional depressives have been found to be statistically comparable at both age of onset and age at index admission. These investigations have used two basic paradigms. The work of Hopkinson (1964) and of Winokur et al. (1980) divided patient samples into early-onset (EO) and late-onset (LO) categories, by using the arbitrarily chosen age of 50 as a cutoff, and compared the groups across a series of clinical variables including delusionality. More recent investigations have focused on delusional depression. These studies divide major depressives into delusional and nondelusional groups and then compare the groups for differences in various indices including age of onset and age at index (Charney and Nelson 1981; Frances et al. 1981; Glassman and Roose 1981). Both paradigms have been carried out in mixed-age samples of adult patients and, therefore, suffer from the same methodologic flaw: Their ability to identify an age effect that occurs only in late life is limited by the broad age range of the samples. Any late-life association between delusions and depression would be washed out by the preponderance of younger adults in the patients studied.

In a study limited to elderly depressives, Post (1982) reported that 37 of 92 such patients (40.2 percent) were delusional. Our own pilot study of 34 elderly endogenous depressives found 19 of these patients (56 percent) to be delusional (Meyers et al. 1984). We also demonstrated a highly significant association between lateness of onset, as defined by first episode at age 60 or later, and the presence of delusions. The present investigation is an extension of our earlier work, in an attempt to clarify the contribution of age factors to the association between delusionality and late-life major depression.

This work was supported in part by grant 5K07MH0043 from the National Institute of Mental Health.

The appropriate treatment of delusional depression remains controversial (Glassman et al. 1975; Nelson and Bowers 1978; Quitkin et al. 1978). To our knowledge, this question has not yet been studied in elderly patients. This report provides information on response to treatment in a subset of our elderly depressives for whom such data has been gathered and analyzed.

METHOD

The records of all patients admitted to the 66 acute psychogeriatric beds of the Westchester Division of The New York Hospital–Cornell University Medical Center, in the five years between January 1, 1979 and December 31, 1983 were reviewed. The charts of patients who met *Diagnostic and Statistical Manual of Mental Disorders, Third Edition* (DSM-III) criteria for a major depressive episode were eligible for inclusion. The depressive illness had to be unipolar and primary. Specific inclusion and exclusion criteria are described in an earlier study (Meyers et al. 1984). Age of onset and delusionality were also determined as previously described. No distinction was made between mood-congruent and -incongruent delusions as long as a major depression was present. Depressive feelings and thoughts such as those of guilt and hopelessness were not considered delusional unless accompanied by a fixed and irrational explanation.

Examination of treatment outcome utilized a naturalistic chart review design. Choice of therapy was made by the patient's physician–therapist in conjunction with the treatment team. General guidelines of the three treatment units involved included: use of a tricyclic antidepressant (TCA) alone for a major depression that was uncomplicated by the presence of delusions or specific medical risk factors; use of a TCA combined with an antipsychotic agent (TCA–AP) or electroconvulsive therapy (ECT) for patients with delusional depression; use of ECT for patients preferring this treatment, for patients not responding to or failing to tolerate medication, and for patients with medical risk factors that would complicate medication treatment.

Only patients who received adequate treatment trials were considered in outcome comparisons. An adequate therapeutic trial was considered as a minimum of eight seizures induced by bilateral ECT or a minimum of three weeks of TCAs at acceptable doses and/or blood levels. Adequate dosage of the tertiary amine TCAs was defined as at least 150 mg per day of amitriptyline, doxepin, or imipramine. Adequate dosage of desipramine or nortriptyline was defined as at least 75 mg per day. Ten-day steady state plasma levels were routinely obtained to ensure appropriateness of dosage.

For the purpose of this report, treatment response was considered dichotomously. Patients who achieved marked improvement or remission were categorized as "much improved"; patients whose charts demonstrated no or only mild improvement were arbitrarily defined as "not improved."

Statistical analysis utilized Student's t-test for continuous data and chi-square analysis with Yates' correction when applicable for dichotomous data.

RESULTS

Age and Delusional Depression

Mean ± SD age at index admission for the 152 patients was 71.7 ± 6.7, and at onset, 56.2 ± 17.3. Sixty-seven of the patients (44 percent) were delusional. Delusional and nondelusional patients did not significantly differ at age of index (72.6 ± 6.8 versus 71 ± 6.5), but delusional patients were highly significantly older at age of onset. Mean age of onset for delusional patients was 63.4 ± 14.6 compared to 50.6 ± 17.3 for nondelusional (t = 4.93, df = 149 p <.001).

Age-of-onset distribution is presented in Table 1, which indicates a tendency for more patients to have their first episodes with increasing age. In 82 cases (54 percent), the first episode was reported as occurring after the sixth decade. As indicated by Table 1, the association between age of onset and delusionality did not become apparent until the seventh decade.

Utilizing the median age of onset of 60 as a cutoff, 17 of the 70 EO patients (24 percent) were delusional compared to 50 of 82 LO patients (61 percent) (χ^2_c = 19.16, p < .001). Examining the data

Table 1. Frequency of Age of Onset and Delusionality by Decade, of 152 Elderly Major Depressives (Separated by Sex)

Age of Onset	Number of Patients			Number (%) Delusional		
	Male	Female	Total	Male	Female	Total
10–19	1	3	4	0	2 (67)	2 (50)
20–29	3	7	10	1 (33)	0	1 (10)
30–39	3	12	15	0	1 (8)	1 (7)
40–49	2	15	17	0	6 (40)	7 (41)
50–59	7	17	24	5 (71)	2 (12)	7 (29)
60–69	13	32	45	8 (62)	15 (47)	23 (51)
70–79	1	29	30	0	22 (76)	22 (73)
80–89	1	6	7	1 (100)	4 (67)	5 (71)

Table 2. Presence of Delusions by Age of Onset in 152 Elderly Major Depressives

	Number (%) Delusional	Number (%) Nondelusional
Onset < 60	17 (25)	53 (62)
Onset > 60	50 (75)	32 (38)
Total	67 (100)	85 (100)

Note. $\chi^2_c = 19.16, p < .001$.

from the perspective of a delusional/nondelusional dichotomy also reveals a highly significant association between delusionality and age of onset (Table 2). In the delusional group, 17 of the 67 patients (25 percent) had an onset of depression prior to age 60, while 50 of the 67 patients (75 percent) had their first episode at age 60 or greater. In the nondelusional group, by contrast, 53 of 85 (62 percent) were EO patients while 32 of 85 (38 percent) were LO patients ($\chi^2_c = 19.16, p < .001$).

Age, Sex and Delusional Depression

Of the 121 women, 52 (43 percent) were delusional compared to 15 of the 31 men (48 percent). A gender effect on the association between age of onset and delusionality was identified. The association occurred earlier in men than in women (Table 1). Five of the seven men (71 percent) having their first episode between 50 and 59 were delusional compared to two of the 17 women (12 percent) with onset during this decade. One of the nine men with onset before age 50 (11 percent) was delusional compared to 14 of the 22 men (64 percent) with onset after this age ($\chi^2_c = 5.11, p < .01$). In women, onset at age 70 discriminated delusional from nondelusional patients: 26 of 86 women (22 percent) having onset before 70 were delusional compared to 26 of 35 (74 percent) with onset at 70 or after ($\chi^2_c = 17.94\ p < .001$).

TREATMENT OUTCOME

Response to treatment was determined in 50 randomly selected delusional depressives and compared with that in 50 nondelusional patients. One of the delusional patients and three of the nondelusionals were discharged without receiving adequate treatment trials. Two nondelusional depressives responded to "inadequate treatment." The treatment of the remaining 49 delusional and 45 nondelusional patients is described in Tables 3 and 4. Twenty-seven of the 49 delusional patients (55 percent) were much improved by their initial treatment. Eighteen of these 28 responders (64 percent) received ECT. Delusional patients who received TCAs alone or in combination with APs had comparably low response rates (36 percent and 29 percent). Combining the two medication treatment groups and comparing the response rate to that of the ECT group demonstrated ECT to be significantly more effective (χ^2_c = 11.84, $p < .001$). Moreover 20 of the 22 delusional patients who did not respond to initial medication treatment subsequently received ECT. Eighteen of these patients (90 percent) responded. Although 13 of the 22 nondelusional depressives (59 percent) responded to adequate trials of TCAs alone, ECT was also the most effective treatment in these patients, with a response rate of 95 percent. The difference in efficacy between ECT and the medication groups was significant (χ^2_c = 4.88, $p < .05$). Although the two forms of medication treatment were more effective in the nondelusional depressives (62 percent) than in the delusionals (32 percent) this difference failed to reach statistical significance (χ^2_c = 3.58, $.1 < p < .2$).

COMMENT

Our finding of delusions in 44 percent of 152 elderly major depressives highlights the importance of this clinical phenomenon. The

Table 3. Initial Treatment Response in 49 Elderly Delusional Depressives

	TCA	TCA–AP	ECT
Much Improved	5 (36)	4 (29)	18 (86)
Not Improved	9 (64)	10 (71)	3 (14)
Total	14 (100)	14 (100)	21 (100)

Note. Data are numbers (%).

Table 4. Initial Treatment Response in 45 Nondelusional Elderly Major Depressives

	TCA	TCA–AP	ECT
Much Improved	13 (59)	3 (75)	18 (95)
Not Improved	9 (41)	1 (25)	1 (5)
Total	22 (100)	4 (100)	19 (100)

Note. Data are numbers (%).

association between delusions and major depression was determined by LO patients. Fifty of the 82 patients (61 percent) with onset after age 60 were delusional compared to 17 of 70 (24 percent) with onset before age 60. Fifty of the 67 delusional patients (75 percent) came from the LO group compared to 32 of the 85 nondelusional patients (38 percent). Delusional and nondelusional patients were of comparable age at index admission. Lateness of onset rather than the effect of aging on previously nondelusional patients caused the association of delusionals and depression in our sample. This conclusion is consistent with the report of Charney and Nelson (1981) that delusionality tends to run true through repeated episodes.

The failure of previous studies to identify this late-life effect results from their use of mixed-age samples of adult patients (Table 5). This strategy can delineate an age correlation that is linear, but would miss a modal association such as that seen in late-onset geriatric conditions (e.g., the dementias and Parkinson's disease).

The treatment of delusional depression can be especially problematic in the elderly. We found that only nine of 28 patients (32 percent) were significantly improved by medication compared to 18 of 21 (86 percent) of those initially treated with ECT. The low rate of medication response is more striking in that careful treatment choice guidelines increased the likelihood of benefit in delusional depressives for whom medication was recommended. When consent was available, the most severely psychotic patients as well as those at greatest medical risk preferentially received ECT. The 86-percent response rate to ECT is similar to that reported for the treatment of depression of mid-life, but is higher than has been suggested for late-life delusional depressions, particularly when patients with marked paranoid features are included (Kantor and Glassman 1977). We suggest this reflects the vigor with which these patients were treated, including the requirement of a minimum of eight seizures induced by bilateral treatments.

None of the ECT patients studied had significant complications. These findings of the efficacy and safety of ECT in the depressed elderly are consistent with recommendations in the literature (Wilson and Major 1972; Fink 1982; Salzman 1982; Raskind 1984).

The 29-percent response rate of delusional depressives to combined treatment is lower than that reported by other investigators (Nelson and Bowers 1978; Minter and Mandel 1979; Kaskey et al. 1980; Spiker et al. 1984). The poor responsiveness did not result from inadequate antidepressant treatment, in that doses and blood levels in our patients were comparable to those utilized with young adults (Meyers and Mei-Tal 1983). However, the limited effectiveness of

Table 5. Age and Delusional Depression

Mean ± SD Age at Onset		Mean ± SD Age Index		
Delusional	Nondelusional	Delusional	Nondelusional	Source
53 ± 10	49 ± 13	59 ± 10	63 ± 7	Glassman and Roose 1981
45.0 ± 14.9	40.1 ± 11.8	54.8 ± 11.8	52.6 ± 14.7	Charney and Nelson 1981
39.5	45.7	57.4	55.1	Frances et al. 1981
63.4 ± 14.6	50.6 ± 17.3*	72.6 ± 6.8	71 ± 6.5	Present study

*$p < .001$.

combined treatment may have resulted from the relatively low doses of antipsychotics used. Elderly patients have been noted to be especially vulnerable to developing parkinsonian side effects to neuroleptics (Ayd 1961; Sovner and DiMascio 1978). This sensitivity may limit the usefulness of combined treatment for elderly delusional depressives.

The retrospective design of this study could have contributed to the results. Although in nearly all cases past history was confirmed by a close relative, delusional patients and their families would be more likely to deny previous episodes. A selection bias could have occurred from EO delusional patients seeking treatment earlier and thereby avoiding hospitalization because of prior experience with a severe illness.

This study did not separate delusion by mood congruence or type. It is therefore unable to address important clinical and investigative issues (Coryell et al. 1984). In younger patients, depressive delusions appear to respond better to antidepressants than do paranoid delusions (Minter and Mandel 1979). Young adult depressives with mood-incongruent delusions are intermediary between schizophrenics and major depressives on measures of short-term outcome and familial pattern (Coryell et al. 1982). The relationship of late-onset delusional depression to other psychiatric entities remains to be explored.

REFERENCES

Ayd FJ Jr: A survey of drug-induced extrapyramidal reactions. JAMA 175:1054–1060, 1961

Charney DS, Nelson JC: Delusional and nondelusional unipolar depression: further evidence for distinct subtypes. Am J Psychiatry 138:328–333, 1981

Coryell W, Tsuang MT, McDaniel J: Psychotic features in major depression: is mood congruence important? J Affective Disord 4:227–236, 1982

Coryell W, Lavori P, Endicott J, et al: Outcome in schizoaffective, psychotic, and nonpsychotic depression. Arch Gen Psychiatry 41:787–791, 1984

Fink M: ECT in the elderly, in Treatment of Psychopathology in the Aging. Edited by Eisdorfer C, Fann WE. New York, Springer, 1982

Frances A, Brown RP, Kocsis JH, et al: Psychotic depression: a separate entity? Am J Psychiatry 138:831–833, 1981

Glassman AH, Roose SP: Delusional depression: a distinct clinical entity? Arch Gen Psychiatry 38:424–427, 1981

Glassman AH, Kantor SJ, Shostak M: Depression, delusions, and drug response. Am J Psychiatry 132:716–719, 1975

Hopkinson G: A genetic study of affective illness in patients over 50. Br J Psychiatry 110:244–254, 1964

Kantor SJ, Glassman AH: Delusional depressions: natural history and response to treatment. Br J Psychiatry 131:351–360, 1977

Kaskey GB, Nasr S, Meltzer HY: Drug treatment in delusional depression. Psychiatry Res 2:267–277, 1980

Meyers BS, Mei-Tal V: Psychiatric reactions during tricyclic treatment of the elderly reconsidered. J Clin Psychopharmacol 3:2–6, 1983

Meyers BS, Kalayam B, Mei-Tal V: Late-onset delusional depression: a distinct clinical entity? J Clin Psychiatry 45:347–349, 1984

Minter RE, Mandel MR: The treatment of psychotic major depressive disorder with drugs and electroconvulsive therapy. J Nerv Ment Dis 167:726–733, 1979

Nelson JC, Bowers MB Jr: Delusional unipolar depression: description and drug response. Arch Gen Psychiatry 35:1321–1328, 1978

Post F: Affective disorders in old age, in Handbook of Affective Disorders. Edited by Paykel E. New York, Guilford Press, 1982

Quitkin F, Rifkin A, Klein DF: Imipramine response in deluded depressive patients. Am J Psychiatry 135:806–811, 1978

Raskind M: Electroconvulsive therapy in the elderly. J Am Geriatr Soc 32:177–178, 1984

Salzman C: A primer on geriatric psychopharmacology. Am J Psychiatry 139:67–74, 1982

Sovner R, DiMascio A: Extrapyramidal syndromes and other neurological side effects of pschyotropic drugs, in Psychopharmacology: A Generation of Progress. Edited by Lipton MA, DiMascio A, Killam KF. New York, Raven Press, 1978

Spiker DG, Griffin S, Cofsky-Weiss J, et al: Pharmacological treatment of delusional depression. Presented at the annual meeting of the American Psychiatric Association, Los Angeles, 1984

Wilson WP, Major LF: Electroshock and the aged patient, in Psychopharmacology and Aging. Edited by Eisdorfer C, Fann WE. New York, Plenum Press, 1972

Winokur G, Behar D, Schlesser M: Clinical and biological aspects of depression in the elderly, in Psychopathology in the Aged. Edited by Cole JO, Barrett JE. New York, Raven Press, 1980

Chapter 3

Outcome of Drug Treatment in Depressed Patients Over the Age of Fifty

Lissy F. Jarvik, M.D., Ph.D.
Sylvia Gerson, Ph.D.

Chapter 3

Outcome of Drug Treatment in Depressed Patients Over the Age of Fifty

Depression appears to be the most common psychiatric disorder among those in the upper age groups. Estimated rates vary over a wide range, depending upon whether they are based on subjective complaints or formal psychiatric evaluation. Blazer (1982), for example, reports prevalence rates in community residents up to 45 percent for symptom checklists, compared to two percent for psychiatric interviews. When it comes to hospital admissions, depressive disorders have been found to account for up to 45 percent of new admissions of persons over the age of 65 to voluntary non-profit and private mental hospitals (Reifler et al. 1982; Turner and Sternberg 1978).

It seems paradoxical that, despite the high frequency of depression among them, persons over the age of 65 years have generally been excluded from treatment-outcome research. Upon reflection, however, it is understandable. Physical illness, medications, susceptibility to side effects, drug–drug and drug–disease interactions all serve to discourage recruitment of geriatric patients for research on the efficacy of pharmacotherapy (Mintz et al. 1981; Weissman and Myers 1979). Hence, in our efforts to locate data on "older" persons, we had to include studies of groups starting as young as age 50, and, in one case, even age 34. And yet, this recently completed search of the literature (Table 1) yielded only 12 double-blind clinical trials in "older" patients (Gerson et al., in press). In eight of these, a tricyclic

---

This work was supported in part by grants MH31357 and MH36205 from the National Institute of Mental Health and by the Veterans Administration.

The opinions expressed in this chapter are those of the authors and are not necessarily those of the Veterans Administration.

Table 1. Previous Drug Treatment Studies with Depressed Patients

Source	Number of patients (beginning/end); Type of Patient	Age (years)	Drug(s)	Dose (mg/day)	Duration
Chesrow et al. 1964	65/61; inpatients	34–87	Nortriptyline	75	7 months
			Placebo		
Kernohan et al. 1967	92/84; inpatients	69 (average)	Nortriptyline	25–100	12 weeks
			Placebo		
Beber 1971	63/60; institution	68–90	Perphenazine/ Amitriptyline	2–8/ 10–40	4 weeks; crossover
			Chlordiazepoxide	10–40	
Zung et al. 1974	36/30; outpatients	60–79	Gerovital	(total, 1,500–2,100)	4 weeks
			Imipramine	62–86	
			Placebo		
Brodie et al. 1975	64/62; outpatients	65 + (average, 73)	Fluphenazine/ Nortriptyline	1.5/30	4 weeks
			Promazine	150	
Olsen et al. 1978	23/21; outpatients	48–77	Gerovital	Week 1: 100 mg 3X/ week; Weeks 2–4: 200 mg 3X/ week	4 weeks of treatment, 1 week off, 4 more weeks of treatment
			Placebo		

Source	Number of patients (beginning/end); Type of Patient	Age (years)	Drug(s)	Dose (mg/day)	Duration
Gerner et al. 1980	60/34; outpatients	60–90	Imipramine Trazodone Placebo	50–200 100–400	4 weeks
Branconnier et al. 1982	75/63; outpatients	60–85	Mianserin Amitriptyline Placebo	30–60 75–150	5 weeks
Goldstein et al. 1982	33/21; institution	64–89	Nomifensine Amitriptyline	75–150 75–150	4 weeks
Scardigli and Jans 1982	87/67 (75 at 2 weeks); inpatients	51–88	Trazodone Nomifensine Mianserin	202–405 75–150 30–60	4 weeks
Branconnier et al. 1983	63/50; inpatients	55–80	Bupropion Imipramine Placebo	150–450 25–150	5 weeks
Jarvik and Mintz, in press	32/9; outpatients	55–81	Imipramine Doxepin Placebo	25–250 25–225	Up to 36 weeks (average, 20 weeks)

antidepressant was one of the test drugs. The tricyclics were amitriptyline, doxepin, imipramine, and nortriptyline. Seven of these trials were placebo-controlled, and the eighth compared amitriptyline with nomifensine (Goldstein et al. 1982). The other four compared the following: trazodone, nomifensine, and mianserin (Scardigli and Jans 1982); gerovital and placebo (Olsen et al. 1978); and combinations of fluphenazine/nortriptyline with promazine (Brodie et al. 1975) or perphenazine/amitriptyline with chlordiazepoxide (Beber 1971). One study included bupropion (Branconnier et al. 1983).

The duration of study treatment was usually four weeks, although one averaged 20 weeks (Jarvik et al. 1982; Jarvik and Mintz, in press); another, 12 weeks (Kernohan et al. 1967); and another, seven months (Chesrow et al. 1964).

Dosages for the tricyclics varied from 25 to 250 mg per day. Blood levels were generally not reported.

The number of subjects varied from 23 to 92 at the beginning of a study, and from nine to 84 at the end. In total, 693 individuals started, and 562 completed the 12 studies. Two of the reports failed to specify the sex of the participants (Brodie et al. 1975; Zung et al. 1974). In the remaining 10, men constituted 43 percent (229 out of 528), a notably higher proportion of men than generally is found among older depressed patients.

In six of the 12 studies, participants were over the age of 60 years, ranging from 60 to 90 years. Three studies accepted patients in their 50s; in one, the range was 48 to 77 years; in another, 34 to 87; and in yet another, only the mean age of 69 years was reported. Taking only the studies with patients all over the age of 60 years, and omitting the two that employed combinations of drugs, we are left with a total of four studies and 148 patients who finished a clinical trial where a tricyclic antidepressant was one of the drugs tested. One of these was a five-week study; the other three lasted four weeks each.

Three of the four studies were placebo-controlled. In all of these, the tricyclic was superior to placebo. In one, trazodone and imipramine showed similar therapeutic efficacy (Gerner et al. 1980). In the other two, mianserin (Branconnier et al. 1982) and gerovital (Zung et al. 1974), led to at least as much improvement as amitriptyline and imipramine, respectively. In another study, however, gerovital produced no significantly greater improvement than placebo (Olsen et al. 1978).

On review, several of the studies suffered from lack of rigorous diagnostic and/or outcome specification (details provided in Gerson et al., in press). Nonetheless, the evidence points to the superiority of tricyclics over placebo. Some of the other antidepressants have fewer side effects than the tricyclics, but data on efficacy are still inadequate. In fact, further data are clearly needed for the tricyclics as well; 148 patients, less than half of whom actually received a tricyclic rather than placebo or comparison drug, is hardly an adequate data base. Data on treatment outcome need to be gathered on patients specified by age, classified with diagnostic rigor, and matched appropriately for sex, severity of illness, and eventually for social supports and psychosocial variables. Treatment course needs to be checked and outcome carefully documented not only during the study but during extended follow-up as well.

REFERENCES

Beber CR: Treating anxiety and depression in the elderly: a double-blind crossover evaluation of two widely used tranquilizers. J Fla Med Assoc 58:35–38, 1971

Blazer DG II: Depression in Late Life. St. Louis, CV Mosby, 1982, pp 103–117

Branconnier RJ, Cole JO, Ghazvinian S, et al: Treating the depressed elderly patient: the comparative behavioral pharmacology of mianserin and amitriptyline, in Typical and Atypical Antidepressants: Clinical Practice. Edited by Costa E, Racagni G. New York, Raven Press, 1982, pp 195–212

Branconnier RJ, Cole JO, Ghazvinian S, et al: Clinical pharmacology of bupropion and imipramine in elderly depressives. J Clin Psychiatry 4:130–133, 1983

Brodie NH, McGhie RL, O'Hara H, et al: Anxiety/depression in elderly patients: a double-blind comparative study of fluphenazine/nortriptyline and promazine. The Practitioner 215:660–664, 1975

Chesrow EJ, Kaplitz SE, Breme JT, et al: Nortriptyline for the treatment of anxiety and depression in chronically ill and geriatric patients. J Am Geriatr Soc 12:271–277, 1964

Gerner R, Estabrook W, Steuer J, et al: Treatment of geriatric depression with trazodone, imipramine, and placebo: a double-blind study. J Clin Psychiatry 41:216–220, 1980

Gerson S, Mintz J, Jarvik LF: Treatment of depression in the elderly, in Perspectives in Psychopharmacology. Edited by Barchas JD, Bunney WE Jr. New York, Alan R Liss (in press)

Goldstein SE, Birnbom F, Laliberte R: Nomifensine in the treatment of depressed geriatric patients. J Clin Psychiatry 43:287–289, 1982

Jarvik LF, Mintz J: Treatment of depression in old age: what works? in Disturbed Behavior in the Elderly. Edited by Awad AG, Durost HB, McCormick WO, et al. Jamaica, NY, SP Medical & Scientific Books, (in press)

Jarvik LF, Mintz J, Steuer J: Treating geriatric depression: a 26-week interim analysis. J Am Geriatr Soc 30:713–717, 1982

Kernohan WJ, Chambers JL, Wilson WT et al: Effects of nortriptyline on the mental and social adjustment of geriatric patients in a mental hospital. J Am Geriatr Soc 15:196–202, 1967

Mintz J, Steuer J, Jarvik LF: Psychotherapy with depressed elderly patients: research considerations. J Consult Clin Psychol 49:542–548, 1981

Olsen EJ, Bank L, Jarvik LF: Gerovital H3: a clinical trial as an antidepressant. J Gerontol 33:514–520, 1978

Reifler BV, Larson E, Hanley R: Coexistence of cognitive impairment and depression in geriatric outpatients. Am J Psychiatry 139:623–626, 1982

Scardigli G, Jans G: Comparative double-blind study on efficacy and side-effects of trazodone, nomifensine, and mianserin in elderly patients. Adv Biochem Psychopharmacol 31:229–237, 1982

Turner RJ, Sternberg MP: Psychosocial factors in elderly patients admitted to a psychiatric hospital. Age Ageing 7:171–177, 1978

Weissman M, Myers J: Depression in the elderly: search directions in psychopathology, epidemiology, and treatment. J Geriatric Psychiatry 12:187–201, 1979

Zung WWK, Gianturco D, Pfeiffer E: Pharmacology of depression in the aged: evaluation of Gerovital-H3 as an antidepressant drug. Psychosomatics 15:127–131, 1974

Chapter 4

Cardiovascular Effects of the Antidepressants: Treating the Elderly Patient

Richard C. Veith, M.D.

Chapter 4

Cardiovascular Effects of the Antidepressants: Treating the Elderly Patient

Because the antidepressants can be cardiotoxic after an overdose, their use has been considered potentially unsafe in some older patients, particularly those with cardiovascular disease. This belief often presents a therapeutic dilemma, since depression is highly prevalent among the elderly and aging is associated with an increased risk of cardiac disease. The reputation of the tri- and tetracyclic antidepressants for cardiotoxicity originally derived from evidence that an overdose can produce marked disturbances in cardiac rhythm and impairment of ventricular conduction (Bigger et al. 1978; Langou et al. 1980). In addition, reports of unexplained sudden death in medically ill patients receiving amitriptyline (Moir et al. 1972) raised concern that these agents might also be cardiotoxic in some patients receiving typical clinical doses. Recent studies have systematically investigated the cardiovascular effects of therapeutic doses of the antidepressants, leading to a clearer understanding of the potential risks of treatment. Nevertheless, lingering concerns persist among clinicians, which may interfere with appropriate treatment provision to the older patient. The purpose of this paper is to review the cardiovascular effects of the tri- and tetracyclic antidepressants and to discuss the clinical implications of these findings in the treatment of the elderly depressed patient.

POTENTIAL EFFECTS OF ANTIDEPRESSANTS ON CARDIOVASCULAR REGULATION

The antidepressants possess a number of pharmacologic properties which should be expected to alter cardiovascular function. The potential effects of the antidepressants on the cardiovascular system can be best appreciated by examining the mechanisms of cardiovascular regulation and the specific pharmacologic profiles of the antidepressants.

Under normal physiologic conditions, heart rate, cardiac rhythm, cardiac output, and blood pressure are carefully controlled by a complex array of counter-regulatory systems involving an interaction between intrinsic cardiac mechanisms and neuroendocrine systems. The sinus node functions as the pacemaker for the heart. Impulses arising in the sinus node initiate atrial contraction and are transmitted to the atrioventricular node, the bundle of His, and the Purkinje fibers, thereby activating a synchronized contraction of the ventricles. Cardiac disease and drugs can interfere with normal sinus pacemaker function, intracardiac electrical conduction, or ventricular contraction, producing changes in heart rate, disturbances in cardiac rhythm, and/or impairment of the intrinsic inotropic effect of the myocardial pumping mechanisms.

It is important to recognize that the heart also receives central nervous system (CNS) neural input via the sympathetic and parasympathetic nervous systems. This CNS input is closely regulated by the vasomotor center in the midbrain, which integrates descending cortical and hypothalamic input, autonomic efferent activity, and afferent feedback from peripheral baroreceptors (Isaac 1980). Impulses transmitted in the sympathetic nerves innervating the heart increase heart rate and increase the force of myocardial contraction. Postganglionic sympathetic neurons also regulate blood pressure by releasing norepinephrine, which stimulates alpha-1 adrenergic receptors on peripheral arteries to produce vasoconstriction. Increased activity of the cholinergic parasympathetic pathways is transmitted to the heart via the vagus nerve and results in a slowing of heart rate.

The antidepressant medications are highly concentrated by cardiac tissues (Weld and Bigger 1980) and possess a number of pharmalogic properties which should be expected to influence normal cardiovascular regulation. The anticholinergic properties of these agents antagonize parasympathetic slowing of heart rate and produce an increase in heart rate. These drugs also have been shown to increase circulating plasma norepinephrine (Veith et al. 1983). This may indicate an increase in sympathetic nervous system outflow or may reflect reduced clearance of plasma norepinephrine. Increased sympathetic stimulation of the heart or activation of cardiac beta adrenergic receptors by circulating norepinephrine could increase heart rate, myocardial automaticity, and cardiac output. To varying degrees, the antidepressants also antagonize peripheral alpha-1 adrenergic receptors (U'Pritchard et al. 1978), which might contribute to the orthostatic blood pressure changes observed in patients taking these medications. In addition, it has been speculated that the antidepressants or their hydroxy metabolites may directly alter cellular electrophysiological properties of myocardial tissues, which may account for their tendency to delay intraventricular conduction (Isaac 1980) and possibly to antagonize myocardial pump function at high concentrations (Young et al. 1984).

ELECTROCARDIOGRAPHIC EFFECTS OF THE ANTIDEPRESSANTS

Recent clinical studies have examined the relationship between plasma levels and electrocardiographic (ECG) effects of the antidepressants following overdose, and in patients receiving therapeutic doses. Petit et al. (1977) and Spiker et al. (1975) investigated the effects of antidepressant overdose on cardiovascular function and found that tricyclic antidepressant levels of ≥1,000 ng/ml were associated with an increased frequency of ventricular rate of ≥120 beats/minute, bundle branch block, cardiac arrhythmias, and cardiac arrest. Prolongation of the QRS interval of >100 msec, present in all patients with plasma levels of >1,000 ng/ml, was a useful clinical indicator of a serious tricyclic antidepressant overdose.

Although there have been few clinical studies of elderly patients or those with known cardiovascular disease, several recent studies have carefully investigated the relationship between therapeutic doses of the antidepressants and their effects on the electrocardiogram (Veith et al. 1980; Veith et al. 1982b; Glassman and Bigger 1981). In young healthy individuals receiving customary outpatient doses of the tri- and tetracyclic antidepressants resulting in plasma levels up to 600 to 800 ng/ml, the antidepressants usually increase heart rate 10 to 15 beats/minute. This is presumably due primarily to an anticholinergic effect. In addition, these agents tend to prolong the PR interval, QRS interval, and QT interval corrected for rate (Veith et al. 1982b). These latter changes are generally not clinically important in healthy patients and do not usually exceed the upper limits of normal for these ECG parameters. The significance of these findings, however, is that they indicate that the antidepressants delay intracardiac conduction.

Using His-bundle electrocardiography, Vohra et al. (1975) have determined that the tricyclic antidepressants delay intraventricular conduction by prolonging transit of electrical impulses through the distal Purkinje specialized conducting system of the ventricles. This effect is reversible, appears to be dose-related and, interestingly, is a property similar to the Class 1-A antiarrhythmics such as quinidine.

Animal studies suggest that the majority of the currently available tri- and tetracyclic antidepressants exhibit this property. Bupropion, an investigational antidepressant not yet available in this country, appears to be less likely than the tricyclic antidepressants to prolong intraventricular conduction (Wenger and Stern 1983).

The few studies performed among elderly individuals or those with cardiovascular disease indicate that the antidepressants produce ECG changes in these populations similar to those observed in young healthy patients (Veith et al. 1982b; Giardina and Bigger 1982). Presumably, patients with pre-existing conduction disturbances and possibly those taking Class 1-A antiarrhythmics might be at increased risk for the development of additional intraventricular conduction delay. However, this possibility has not been systematically examined in clinical studies (Glassman and Bigger 1981).

EFFECTS ON CARDIAC RHYTHM

Until the late 1970s, it was widely believed that even in therapeutic doses, the tricyclic antidepressants were likely to induce arrhythmias in patients with cardiovascular disease. However, as noted above, clinical and animal studies suggest that these agents produce a "quinidine-like" effect on intraventricular conduction. In the 1970s, Wilkerson (1978) demonstrated that the tricyclic antidepressants effectively prevented experimentally induced cardiac arrhythmias in doses comparable to and slightly above those used clinically. Bigger and associates (1977) subsequently demonstrated a reduction in premature ventricular contractions in two patients treated with imipramine. Veith et al. (1982a) confirmed the antiarrhythmic effect of imipramine in depressed patients selected for the presence of heart disease who had a prior history of myocardial infarction and/or coronary artery by-pass surgery. In the most convincing demonstration of the antiarrhythmic effects of imipramine, Giardina and Bigger (1982) demonstrated greater than an 80 percent reduction in premature ventricular complexes, bigeminy, and ventricular tachycardia in 22 cardiac patients without clinical psychological depression who received between 100 and 300 mg of imipramine per day. Interestingly, 64 percent of these patients had previously failed to respond adequately to customary antiarrhythmic drug treatment.

Of the currently available antidepressant agents, therapeutic doses of imipramine (Veith et al. 1982a; Giardina and Bigger 1982; Bigger et al. 1977), nortriptyline (Giardina et al. 1981), and maprotiline (Raeder et al. 1979) have been shown by continuous electrocardiographic monitoring to effectively reduce ventricular dysrhythmias. Careful examination of electrocardiographic and electrophysiologic data from human and animal studies suggests that all of the currently available tri- and tetracyclic antidepressants should share this property, although there may be differences in potency among various agents. In contrast, trazodone may actually increase ventricular dysrhythmias according to a recent case report (Janowski et al. 1983). Further controlled studies are required to confirm this clinical impression.

EFFECTS ON MYOCARDIAL PERFORMANCE

Although studies in animals have shown a direct myocardial depressant effect by tricyclic antidepressants, this effect appears to occur in plasma concentrations that are in the toxic range for human beings (Veith 1982). Studies of systolic time intervals (simultaneous recording of the ECG, phonocardiogram, and carotid pulse wave) in adults receiving therapeutic doses of antidepressants have suggested that myocardial contractility is reduced (Taylor and Braithwaite 1978; Kopera 1980; Raeder 1978; Burckhardt 1978; Burgess 1978). However, systolic time intervals are indirect measurements that can be influenced by factors other than changes in ventricular performance (for example, sex, age, heart rate, blood pressure, or bundle branch block) (Swain et al. 1980). Thus, changes in systolic time intervals, interpreted as evidence of an antidepressant-induced negative inotropic effect, may instead simply reflect the prolongation of the intraventricular conduction that is commonly observed with these agents.

More recent studies have used a sensitive and reliable radionuclide technique to assess the effects of antidepressant therapy on ventricular function. Veith et al. (1982a) found no adverse effect of therapeutically effective doses of imipramine and doxepin on measurements of the left ventricular ejection fraction in depressed patients with cardiac disease. This finding was confirmed by Glassman et al. (1983) who studied cardiac patients with even more severely impaired left ventricular pump function. Although these studies indicate that customary therapeutic doses of the tricyclic antidepressants appear to have no clinically important effect on left ventricular pump function, it should not be concluded that antidepressant treatment of patients with impaired ventricular function is without hazards. Both studies found that cardiac patients may be at particular risk for the development of postural hypotension from these agents. In addition, patients with cardiac disease who achieve unusually high plasma concentrations of the antidepressants or their hydroxy metabolites (Young et al. 1984) would be the most susceptible to any negative inotropic effects of these agents.

EFFECTS ON BLOOD PRESSURE

Although the tricyclic antidepressants occasionally cause a modest increase in supine systolic blood pressure, more commonly these drugs produce postural hypotension. Numerous studies suggest that more than 20 percent of patients receiving these agents will experience this adverse effect (Glassman and Bigger 1981; Veith et al. 1982b; Glassman et al. 1983; Glassman et al. 1979). Although early studies emphasized that postural hypotension may be a particular risk for the elderly, Glassman et al. (1979) found no relationship between imipramine-induced orthostatic hypotension and such factors as age, dose, the presence of preexisting heart disease, or the plasma-imipramine concentration. They found that the best predictor of orthostatic hypotension during imipramine treatment was the degree of orthostatic hypotension prior to treatment.

As noted above, patients with cardiac disease appear to be especially susceptible for the development of this adverse effect. Glassman et al. (1983) found that seven of 15 patients with cardiac disease developed severe orthostatic hypotension during treatment with imipramine. Similarly, Veith et al. (1982a) showed that four of 17 cardiac patients receiving imipramine or doxepin developed either symptomatic orthostasis or syncopy during treatment. These studies indicate the need for particular caution when using the agents in patients with heart disease or those concomitantly treated with drugs that reduce blood pressure, such as the antihypertensives or oral nitrates.

The relative importance of such factors as antidepressant dose, the presence of heart disease, and specific drug selection in accounting for the development of postural hypotension remains unclear. Two studies have suggested that nortriptyline is less likely than imipramine to produce orthostasis (Roose et al. 1979; Thayssen et al. 1981). However, in both studies, plasma levels were substantially lower in patients who received nortriptyline. Thus, it may be the lower optimal plasma levels recommended for nortriptyline rather than an inherent pharmacologic difference from other tricyclic antidepressants which accounts for the apparent advantage of using nortriptyline in high-risk patients. Promising evidence does suggest that in therapeutically effective doses, bupropion is much less likely than imipramine to produce orthostatic hypotension (Farid et al. 1983). Because this agent is also not anticholinergic, it may ultimately be advantageous in the treatment of older patients.

CARDIOVASCULAR EFFECTS OF THE MAO INHIBITORS AND LITHIUM CARBONATE

Although the cardiovascular effects of the monoamine oxidase (MAO) inhibitors and lithium carbonate have not been widely investigated, several aspects of their use in elderly patients deserve attention. Robinson et al. (1982) have shown that, unlike the tricyclic and tetracyclic antidepressants, the MAO inhibitor phenelzine tends to decrease heart rate and to shorten the QT interval corrected for rate. As with the tricyclic antidepressants, clinically effective doses of the MAO inhibitors routinely produce orthostatic hypotension. The degree of orthostatic hypotension appears to be correlated with the degree of inhibition of monoamine oxidase. Combined with the potential difficulties in dietary compliance, the propensity to produce orthostatic hypotension greatly complicates the use of MAO inhibitors in older patients.

Generally, lithium has little effect on cardiovascular function or blood pressure. However, it has been reported that older individuals can develop bradycardia and sinus node dysfunction during lithium treatment (Roose et al. 1979). Because this may occur in patients with occult cardiovascular disease, it has been recommended that the electrocardiogram be routinely monitored when initiating lithium treatment in older patients.

IMPLICATIONS FOR TREATING THE ELDERLY

Because recent studies have more carefully characterized the cardiovascular effects of antidepressant treatment, it is now possible to more specifically define the risks of treatment for older individuals or those with cardiovascular disease. The increase in heart rate observed with these agents might be poorly tolerated by patients with significant ischemic heart disease or uncontrolled angina, for whom an increase in heart rate may further compromise cardiac oxygenation. Although the effect of the tricyclic antidepressants to increase plasma norephinephrine levels might promote ventricular irritability, it increasingly appears that the predominant effect of the majority of these drugs on cardiac rhythm is a membrane-stabilizing, antiarrhythmic effect. However, the tendency of the antidepressants to prolong intracardiac conduction requires that special care be exercised in treating patients with preexisting conduction disturbances or those receiving concomitant Class 1-A antiarrhythmic agents such as quinidine or pronestyl. Should an arrhythmia or conduction disturbance develop during antidepressant treatment, the drug should be stopped if the disturbance is deemed clinically significant. Electroconvulsive therapy, which is safe and effective in cardiac patients, or the use of MAO inhibitors, which do not delay intraventricular conduction, might be considered as alternative treatments. The emergence of clinically insignificant ECG alterations would generally not preclude continued antidepressant therapy. Because trazodone has been implicated in the development of ventricular dysrhythmias, this agent should be avoided or used with particular caution in patients with cardiac disease.

Orthostatic hypotension is particularly hazardous for the elderly, for whom complications from trauma and falls may be catastrophic. This risk may be reduced with careful monitoring of pretreatment postural hypotension and cautious treatment (i.e., starting with low doses, progressing slowly, using divided doses, and avoiding high doses if possible). Nortriptyline may offer a selective advantage in the treatment of high-risk patients because of its relatively well-established optimal blood level range within which patients appear to be less likely to develop orthostatic hypotension. Bupropion may ultimately be advantageous in treating elderly patients, because of its lack of anticholinergic effects and its reduced likelihood for prolonging intracardiac conduction and producing orthostatic hypotension.

Treatment of older or frail patients can generally begin with 25 to 50 mg of the selected agent, increasing in 25-mg increments at three- to five-day intervals, using divided doses when 100 mg just before sleep is exceeded. Supine and standing blood pressure should be measured prior to treatment and monitored regularly during treatment. A pretreatment electrocardiogram should be obtained to identify patients with preexisting conduction disturbances or those with unstable arrhythmias. In patients considered at high risk for the development of conduction disturbances or other cardiovascular adverse effects, the electrocardiogram should be repeated during treatment, recognizing that five to seven days may be required to achieve steady-state plasma levels following a dosing increment.

With the exception of nortriptyline, for which optimal plasma levels appear to fall within the 50 to 150 ng/ml range, the relationship between plasma antidepressant levels and therapeutic efficacy are not well established (Friedel 1982). In addition, studies indicate only a modest relationship between plasma antidepressant levels and electrocardiographic or blood pressure changes (Veith et al. 1980; Veith et al. 1982b; Glassman and Bigger 1981; Glassman et al. 1979). Thus, there is little clinical value in routinely monitoring plasma antidepressant levels.

Particular caution should be exercised in using antidepressants in the following clinical circumstances: 1) within the immediate recovery period of a myocardial infarction or any other significant change in cardiovascular function, until cardiovascular function has stabilized; 2) in patients with poorly controlled ventricular arrhythmias, uncontrolled angina, or poorly compensated congestive heart failure; 3) in patients with pre-existing first-degree heart block or bundle branch block (treatment MAO inhibitors or ECT may provide useful alternatives); and 4) in patients with significant pretreatment postural hypotension or those taking other drugs that reduce blood pressure.

REFERENCES

Bigger JT Jr, Giardina EGV, Perel JM, et al: Cardiac antiarrhythmic effect of imipramine hydrochloride. N Engl J Med 296:206–208, 1977

Bigger JT Jr, Kantor SJ, Glassman AH, et al: Cardiovascular effects of tricyclic antidepressant drugs, in Psychopharmacology: A Generation of Progress. Edited by Lipton MA, DiMascio A, Killam AF. New York, Raven Press, 1978

Burckhardt D, Raeder E, Muller V, et al: Cardiovascular effects of tricyclic and tetracyclic antidepressants. JAMA 239:213–216, 1978

Burgess CD, Turner P, Wadsworth J: Cardiovascular responses to mianserin hydrochloride: a comparison with tricyclic antidepressant drugs. Br J Clin Pharmacol 5:21s–28s, 1978

Farid FF, Wenger TL, Tsai SY, et al: Use of bupropion in patients who exhibit orthostatic hypotension on tricyclic antidepressants. J Clin Psychiatry 44:170–173, 1983

Friedel RO: The relationship of therapeutic response to antidepressant plasma levels: an update. J Clin Psychiatry 43:37–42, 1982

Giardina EGV, Bigger JT Jr: Antiarrhythmic effect of imipramine hydrochloride in patients with ventricular premature complexes without psychological depression. Am J Cardiol 50:172–179, 1982

Giardina EGV, Bigger JT Jr, Johnson LL: The effect of imipramine and nortriptyline on ventricular premature depolarizations and left ventricular function. Circulation 65:316, 1981 (abstr)

Glassman AH, Bigger JT Jr: Cardiovascular effects of therapeutic doses of tricyclic antidepressants: a review. Arch Gen Psychiatry 38:815–820, 1981

Glassman AH, Bigger JT Jr, Giardina EGV, et al: Clinical characteristics of imipramine-induced orthostatic hypotension. Lancet 1:468–472, 1979

Glassman AH, Johnson LL, Giardina EGV, et al: The use of imipramine in depressed patients with congestive heart failure. JAMA 250:1997–2001, 1983

Isaac L: Clonidine in the central nervous system: site and mechanism of hypotensive action. J Cardiovasc Pharmacol 2:S5–S19, 1980

Janowski D, Curtis G, Zisook S, et al: Ventricular arrhythmias possibly aggravated by trazodone. Am J Psychiatry 140:796–797, 1983

Kopera H, Fluch N, Harpf H, et al: Cardiovascular effects of mianserin—a comparative study with amitriptyline and a placebo in healthy subjects. Int J Clin Pharmacol Ther Toxicol 18:104–109, 1980

Langou RA, Van Dyke C, Tahan SR, et al: Cardiovascular manifestations of tricyclic antidepressant overdose. Am Heart J 100:458–464, 1980

Moir DC, Cornwell WB, Dingwall-Fordyce I, et al: Cardiotoxicity of amitriptyline. Lancet 2:561–564, 1972

Petit JM, Spiker DG, Ruwitch JF, et al: Tricyclic antidepressant overdose: clinical presentation and plasma levels. Clin Pharmacol Ther 21:47–51, 1977

Raeder EA, Burckhardt D, Neubauer H, et al: Long-term tri- and tetracyclic antidepressants, myocardial contractility, and cardiac rhythm. Br Med J 2:666–667, 1978

Raeder EA, Zinsli M, Burckhardt D: Effect of maprotiline on cardiac arrhythmias. Br Med J 2:102, 1979

Robinson DS, Nies A, Corcella J, et al: Cardiovascular effects of phenelzine and amitriptyline in depressed outpatients. J Clin Psychiatry 43:8–15, 1982

Roose SP, Nurnberger JI, Dunner DL, et al: Cardiac sinus node dysfunction during lithium treatment. Am J Psychiatry 136:804–806, 1979

Roose SP, Glassman AH, Siris SG, et al: Comparison of imipramine- and nortriptyline-induced orthostatic hypotension: a meaningful difference. J Clin Psychopharmacol 1:316–319, 1981

Spiker DB, Weiss AN, Chang SS, et al: Tricyclic antidepressant overdose: clinical presentation and plasma levels. Clin Pharmacol Ther 18:539–546, 1975

Swain JL, Morris KG, Bruno FP, et al: Comparison of multigated radionuclide angiography with ultrasonic sonomicrometry over a wide range of ventricular function in the conscious dog. Am J Cardiol 46:976–982, 1980

Taylor DJE, Braithwaite RA: Cardiac effects of tricyclic antidepressant medication: a preliminary study of nortriptyline. Br Heart J 40:1005–1009, 1978

Thayssen P, Bjerre M, Kragh-Sorensen P, et al: Cardiovascular effects of imipramine and nortriptyline in elderly patients. Psychopharmacology 74:360–364, 1981

U'Pritchard DC, Greenberg DA, Sheehan PP, et al: Tricyclic antidepressants: therapeutic properties and affinity for alpha-noradrenergic receptor binding sites in the brain. Science 199:197–199, 1978

Veith RC: Cardiac effects of the tricyclic antidepressants: clinical implications for treating the elderly, in Treatment of Psychopathology in the Aging. Edited by Eisdorfer CE, Fann WE. New York, Springer, 1982

Veith RC, Friedel RO, Bloom V, et al: Electrocardiogram changes and plasma desipramine levels during treatment of depression. Clin Pharmacol Ther 27:796–802, 1980

Veith RC, Raskind MA, Caldwell JH, et al: Cardiovascular effects of tricyclic antidepressants in depressed patients with chronic heart disease. N Engl J Med 306:954–959, 1982a

Veith RC, Bloom V, Bielski R, et al: ECG effects of comparable plasma concentrations of desipramine and amitriptyline. J Clin Psychopharmacol 2:394–398, 1982b

Veith RC, Raskind MA, Barnes RF, et al: Tricyclic antidepressants and supine, standing, and exercise plasma norepinephrine levels. Clin Pharmacol Ther 33:763–769, 1983

Vohra J, Burrows G, Hunt D, et al: The effect of toxic and therapeutic doses of tricyclic antidepressant drugs on intracardiac conduction. European Journal of Cardiology 3:219–227, 1975

Weld FM, Bigger JT Jr: Electrophysiological effects of imipramine on ovine cardiac Purkinje and ventricular muscle fibers. Circ Res 46:167–175, 1980

Wenger TL, Stern WC: The cardiovascular profile of bupropion. J Clin Psychiatry 44:176–182, 1983

Wilkerson, RD: Antiarrhythmic effects of tricyclic antidepressant drugs in ouabain-induced arrhythmias in the dog. J Pharmacol Exp Ther 205:666–674, 1978

Young RC, Alexopoulos GS, Shamoian CA, et al: Heart failure associated with high plasma 10-hydroxynortriptyline levels. Am J Psychiatry 141:432–433, 1984

Chapter 5

Psychopharmacologic Treatment of Depression in Elderly Patients with Cardiovascular Disease

James E. Spar, M.D.

Chapter 5

Psychopharmacologic Treatment of Depression in Elderly Patients with Cardiovascular Disease

Psychopharmacologic treatment of elderly depressed patients is often complicated by chronic and acute cardiovascular disease, the presence of which can increase vulnerability to side effects and adverse reactions from antidepressant medications. This chapter will review selected clinical studies and case reports that focus on the actions of non–tricyclic antidepressant medications which pose significant hazard for elderly patients with cardiovascular disease, and then will summarize and propose specific recommendations for treatment of elderly patients with depression and cardiovascular illness.

TRICYCLIC ANTIDEPRESSANTS

The effect of tricyclic antidepressants on the cardiovascular system will not be reviewed here since they are discussed in detail in Chapter 4 by Veith.

MONOAMINE OXIDASE INHIBITORS

By comparison with the tricyclic antidepressants, relatively few studies of the cardiovascular effects of monoamine oxidase inhibitors have been published. Robinson et al. (1981) administered 60 mg/day of phenelzine to 70 outpatients and observed a decline in mean heart rates (from 73 to 67) and mean Qtc intervals (from 432 to 413 msec), and no effect upon QRS intervals. White et al. (1983) observed no effects upon cardiac conduction and a similar decline in heart rate in 10 adults who were treated with tranylcypramine, at an average dosage of 36 mg/day. Four of the patients in this study developed nonspecific T-wave abnormalities, and one developed ventricular premature contractions (four per minute) while on tranylcypramine. Monoamine oxidase inhibitors also cause postural hypotension, the mechanism of which remains incompletely understood.

Kronig et al. (1983) followed 14 patients, of average age 52, who were treated with phenelzine (65 mg/day) and found that the mean orthostatic drop in blood pressure increased with time and peaked (at a maximum mean of 12 mm Hg) between three and four weeks after medications were started. Interestingly, a mean drop in lying systolic pressure of 12 mm Hg also occurred, a finding that is consistent with the original use of monoamine oxidase inhibitors as antihypertensive agents.

LITHIUM

Lithium treatment has long been associated with nonspecific T-wave abnormalities (Demers and Heninger 1971), which have been postulated to occur because of displacement of intracellular cations (including potassium) by the lithium ion, resulting in abnormal repolarization. In general, these changes are benign, reverse with cessation of treatment, and have not been regarded as of significant concern with respect to the administration of lithium to elderly patients. Similarly, although other complications of lithium therapy including myocarditis (Tseng 1971) and ventricular arrhythmia (Tangedahl 1972) have been reported, they appear to be quite rare and have not made a significant impact upon clinical practice. A potentially more disturbing effect of lithium therapy, however, has been emphasized in recent reports. Roose et al. (1981) described three cases of lithium-induced cardiac sinus node dysfunction, bringing to five the number of such cases reported through 1981 (Wellens et al. 1975; Wilson et al. 1976). Roose et al.'s patients were ages 69, 75, and 57; each was asymptomatic and two became dysfunctional on normal therapeutic serum levels of lithium. Each patient developed sinus slowing (with rates as low as 35) and junctional escape beats. These reports raise the possibility that silent but potentially dangerous disturbances of sinus node function may be more common than is generally appreciated.

Lithium therapy may also be complicated by the presence of congestive heart failure, if kidney function is impaired. As lithium is cleared by the kidney, significant reduction of kidney function may result in a dangerous elevation of the serum lithium level (Gershon and Shopsin 1973).

PSYCHOSTIMULANTS

All agents in this category (which includes amphetamines, methylphenidate, magnesium pemoline, and other agents) are capable of producing significant sympathomimetic stimulation of the cardiovascular system, with increases in systolic and diastolic blood pressure, usually accompanied by increases in heart rate. In some cases reflex slowing of heart rate may occur. Methylphenidate, a synthetic amphetamine-like agent with significantly weaker peripheral effects than amphetamine (Perel and Dayton 1977) has received the most attention in the affective disorder literature. Significant cardiovascular stimulation was observed by Janowsky et al. (1978a and 1978b) who administered 0.5 mg/kilogram of methylphenidate intravenously to 17 psychiatric inpatients and recorded a mean increase in systolic blood pressure from 123 to 132, and in diastolic blood pressure from 80 to 89. All cardiovascular effects peaked by 30 minutes following infusion. However, reduced cardiovascular potency associated with oral administration was documented by Crook et al. (1977), who administered 10-mg and 30-mg oral dosages of methylphenidate to 12 subjects (mean age, 72) and observed no changes in heart rate or blood pressure at 30, 60, or 90 minutes following ingestion. Following the administration of an oral dose of 45 mg to eight of the subjects, however, two experienced increased heart rate and blood pressure; in one subject heart rate increased from 80 at baseline to 120 within one hour of drug ingestion. These studies suggest that, in modest oral doses, methylphenidate should be well tolerated by elderly patients, but that extra caution should be used when hypertension or tachyarrhythmia is present.

SECOND-GENERATION ANTIDEPRESSANTS

There are three agents in this category, so called because they are the first antidepressants released in the United States within the past two decades that are not merely newer derivatives of well-known tricyclic agents. They are amoxapine, a dibenzoxazapine derivative closely related to loxapine, a high-potency neuroleptic; maprotiline, a tetracyclic with pharmacologic properties similar to the secondary tricyclics (desmethylimipramine and nortriptyline); and trazodone, a triazolopyridine derivative. Each of these agents has been claimed, based upon animal and early human studies, to be relatively free of the cardiovascular effects of tricyclics. However, as the use of these agents becomes more widespread, the clinical literature is beginning to reflect more cardiovascular effects than were anticipated.

Amoxapine

This agent, the desmethyl derivative of loxapine, was initially reported to have few cardiac side effects, and systematic studies to the contrary have not been published. Published studies do suggest that mild increases in heart rate, probably due to anticholinergic effects, can be expected, but there remains little evidence yet that amoxapine delays or otherwise affects cardiac conduction (Smith and Ayd 1981). However, two recent case reports suggest that amoxapine may possess a poorly understood ability to provoke supraventricular arrhythmia. In one case, atrial flutter developed in an elderly patient with pre-existing heart disease (Zavodnick 1981). The second case was somewhat more ominous; a 69-year-old woman without heart disease (except nonspecific T-wave abnormalities on electrocardiogram) developed frequent premature atrial contractions with trigeminy that were clearly related to administration of amoxapine at a dosage of 250 mg/day. The arrhythmia was responsive to dosage reduction but not to administration of propranalol (Ortiz and Josef 1983). The clinical implications of these reports remain to be determined, but in the meantime, a somewhat increased "index of concern" seems justified when administering amoxapine to elderly patients.

Maprotiline

This agent, which is predominantly a blocker of norepinephrine reuptake in presynaptic axon terminals, has also enjoyed an early "clean bill of health" in regard to its cardiovascular side effects. Gwirtsman et al. (1983) studied 24 patients, having a mean age of 63, who received an average of 144 mg of maprotiline for up to six weeks. The only cardiovascular side effect was orthostatic hypotension, which was observed in 6.6 percent of the patients. Electrocardiograms were performed before and after treatment, but the data were not reported.

Edwards and Goldie (1983) studied 10 subjects, of average age 35, who received 225 mg of maprotiline (one subject received 150 mg). They found a mean increase in heart rate of 22 beats/minute and a mean increase in PR interval from .14 to .16, along with a slight decline in Qtc interval. No changes in the QRS complex or T waves were seen. Electrocardiographic changes did not correlate with plasma drug levels, and the authors concluded that maprotiline does not have quinidine-like effects at therapeutic dosages. However, a recent case report by Herrmann et al. (1983) described QT prolongation and ventricular tachycardia in an 81-year-old woman who was treated with 62.5 mg/day of maprotiline, in combination with several other medications. In this patient electrocardiographic normalization paralleled decline in maprotiline serum levels (which peaked at 169 mg/ml), and the authors concluded with a recommendation that "physicians prescribing maprotiline maintain the same vigilance for cardiovascular side effects as that currently accorded tricyclic antidepressant drugs."

Trazodone

On the basis of animal studies and early human trials this agent was proposed as an ideal treatment for patients with pre-existing cardiac conduction disturbance, who are most likely to develop complete heart block if treated with tricyclic antidepressants. Gomoll et al. (1979) administered trazodone to dogs in amounts equivalent to three to five times recommended therapeutic dosages and failed to observe consistent effects on atrioventricular conduction. Studies in humans, conducted by Mann et al. (1981) in young adults, and Branconnier and Cole (1981) and Hayes et al. (1983) in elderly patients, supported Gomoll et al.'s and other animal studies in finding no significant effects of trazodone on cardiac conduction. Himmelhoch et al. (1984) studied 46 depressed patients, of average age 58, who had varying degrees of chronic heart disease and were described as "fragile, debilitated, and difficult to treat." Dosages varied and an overall mean was not reported, but can be calculated at approximately 200 mg/day. There were no changes in mean PR, QRS, or QT interval, and no instances of exacerbation of pre-existing conduction disturbance. These results were supported by a similar study conducted by Van de Merwe et al. (1984) who concluded that "Trazodone . . . has minimal effects on cardiac conduction over time." Several recent case reports illustrate the potential consequences of even "minimal" effects. Irwin and Spar (1983) reported a case of apparently trazodone-dose-dependent reversible first degree block in a 74-year-old man who was also receiving therapeutic dosages of digitalis. A significantly more alarming case was reported by Rausch et al. (1984), who described a 77-year-old man who developed complete heart block following one 50-mg oral dose of trazodone. Despite these case reports, the bulk of evidence supports the view that trazodone is significantly safer than tricyclic antidepressants in this regard.

Trazodone does not apparently increase heart rate, in keeping with claims that it lacks anticholinergic effects. Hayes et al. (1983) reported no mean increase in heart rate in 20 elderly depressed patients, while Himmelhoch et al. (1984) observed a mean decrease in heart rate of five beats/minute. Significantly, four of Himmelhoch et al.'s patients who had low baseline heart rates became "lightheaded" during treatment with trazodone. This tendency to produce slowing of heart rate was also described by Van de Merwe et al. (1984), who reported a "significant bradycardia" in six young adults who received 300 mg/day of trazodone.

Janowsky et al. (1983) reported two cases of apparent trazodone-induced exacerbation of ventricular arrhythmia, but Himmelhoch et al. (1984, 61), applying strict criteria for worsening, concluded that "while it is possible that there exists some subset of patients upon whom trazodone has an arrhythmogenic effect, it is clear that such effect is, at worst, limited to a small percentage of the treated population."

Finally, trazodone does appear to cause orthostatic decline in blood pressure, as reported by Himmelhoch et al. (1984). However, it appears to be somewhat less potent than tricyclics in this regard, as only three of 46 subjects developed postural hypotension (defined as a 15-mm Hg or more drop in systolic, or 10-mm Hg or more drop in diastolic, pressure), and nine subjects who had pretreatment orthostatic hypotension did not get worse during treatment.

SUMMARY AND TREATMENT RECOMMENDATIONS

The preceding review of selected articles can be summarized as follows:

Monoamine oxidase inhibitors do not appear to influence cardiac conduction; do not increase and may decrease heart rate; and cause postural decline in blood pressure that increases over the first three weeks of treatment, is dose-dependent, and may slightly attenuate over time.

Lithium causes benign T-wave changes and may exert inhibitory effects on sinoatrial node function, but is otherwise relatively free of cardiac effects.

Psychostimulants can increase systolic and diastolic blood pressure and heart rate. Methylphenidate has little effect on heart rate or blood pressure at oral dosages below 45 mg, but a profound effect if administered intravenously.

Second-generation antidepressants appear to be somewhat less free of cardiac effects than initially claimed. Specifically, amoxapine may increase heart rate and, in rare cases, provide supraventricular arrhythmias; maprotiline has cardiac effects similar to tricyclics, increasing heart rate and cardiac conduction time; and trazodone appears to slow heart rate and cause orthostatic hypotension, and may have tricyclic-like effects on cardiac conduction in rare individuals.

Accordingly, the following guidelines are proposed.

1. All elderly patients should be evaluated for cardiovascular illness prior to initiation of antidepressant therapy. A cardiovascular history, physical examination, determination of postural change in blood pressure, and 12-lead electrocardiogram are recommended.

2. Monoamine oxidase inhibitors
   a. Should be prescribed *with caution* for patients with bradyarrhythmias or hypotension.
   b. Patients should be instructed to rise from a seated position slowly, preferably while stabilizing posture by holding on to a stable support, while under treatment.
   c. Routine daily determinations of orthostatic change in blood pressure are recommended for hospitalized patients.
3. Lithium
   a. Should not be prescribed for patients with bradyarrhythmia or "sick sinus" syndrome.
   b. Should be prescribed *with caution* for patients with ventricular arrhythmia or congestive heart failure.
4. Psychostimulants
   Should be prescribed *with caution* in patients with tachyarrhythmia or hypertension.
5. Second-generation antidepressants
   a. Maprotiline should be regarded as essentially similar to tricyclic antidepressants, perhaps most comparable to desmethylimipramine.
   b. Amoxapine should be prescribed *with caution* for patients with tachyarrhythmia, angina pectoris, or supraventricular arrhythmia.
   c. Trazodone should be prescribed *with caution* for patients with bradyarrhythmia or ventricular arrhythmia.

REFERENCES

Branconnier RJ, Cole JO: Effects of acute administration of trazodone and amitriptyline on cognition, cardiovascular function, and salivation in the normal geriatric subject. J Clin Psychopharmacol 1(Suppl):82s–88s, 1981

Crook T, Ferris S, Sathananthan G, et al: The effect of methylphenidate on test performance in the cognitively impaired aged. Psychopharmacology 52:251–255, 1977

Demers R, Heninger G: Electrocardiographic T-wave changes during lithium carbonate treatment. JAMA 218:381–386, 1971

Edwards JG, Goldie A: Mianserin, maprotiline and intracardiac conduction. Br J Clin Pharmacol 15:249s–254s, 1983

Gershon S, Shopsin B: Lithium: Its Role in Psychiatric Research and Treatment. New York, Plenum Press, 1973, p 171

Gomoll AW, Byrne JE, Deitchman D: Hemodynamic and cardiac actions of trazodone and imipramine in the anesthetized dog. Life Sci 24:1841–1848, 1979

Gwirtsman HE, Ahles S, Halaris A, et al: Therapeutic superiority of maprotiline versus doxepin in geriatric depression. J Clin Psychiatry 44:449–453, 1983

Hayes RL, Gerner RH, Fairbanks L, et al: ECG findings in geriatric depressives given trazodone, placebo or imipramine. J Clin Psychiatry 44:180–183, 1983

Herrmann HC, Kaplan LM, Bierer BE: Q-T prolongation and torsades de pointes ventricular tachycardia produced by the tetracyclic antidepressant agent maprotiline. Am J Cardiol 51:904–906, 1983

Himmelhoch JM, Schechtman K, Auchenbach R: The role of trazodone in the treatment of depressed cardiac patients. Psychopathology 17(Suppl 2):51–63, 1984

Irwin M, Spar JE: Reversible cardiac condition abnormality associated with trazodone administration (letter). Am J Psychiatry 140:945–946, 1983

Janowsky D, Curtis G, Zisook S, et al: Ventricular arrhythmias possibly aggravated by trazodone. Am J Psychiatry 140:796–797, 1983

Janowsky DS, Leichner P, Parker D, et al: The effect of methylphenidate on serum growth hormone. Influence of antipsychotic drugs and diagnosis. Arch Gen Psychiatry 35:1384–1389, 1978a

Janowsky DS, Leichner P, Parker D, et al: Methylphenidate and serum prolactin in man. Psychopharmacology 58:43–57, 1978b

Kronig MH, Roose SP, Walsh BT, et al: Blood pressure effects of phenelzine. J Clin Psychopharmacol 3:307, 1983

Mann JJ, Georgotas A, Newton R, et al: A controlled study of trazodone, imipramine, and placebo in outpatients with endogenous depression. J Clin Psychopharmacol 1:75–80, 1981

Ortiz A, Josef NC: Premature atrial contractions and amoxapine therapy: a case report. J Clin Psychopharmacol 3:246–249, 1983

Perel JM, Dayton PG: Methylphenidate, in Psychotherapeutic Drugs—Part II: Applications. Edited by Usdin E, Forrest IS. New York, Marcel Dekker, 1977, pp 1287–1316

Rausch JL, Pavlinac DM, Newman PE: Complete heart block following a single dose of trazodone. Am J Psychiatry 141:1472–1473, 1984

Robinson DS, Corcella J, Nies A, et al: Cardiovascular effects of amitriptyline and phenelzine. Clin Pharmacol Ther 29:276–277, 1981

Roose SP, Nurnberger JI, Dunner DL, et al: Cardiac sinus node dysfunction during lithium treatment. Am J Psychiatry 136:804–806, 1979

Smith RS Jr, Ayd FJ Jr: A critical appraisal of amoxapine. J Clin Psychiatry 42 (6):238–242, 1981

Tangedahl T, Gau G: Myocardial irritability associated with lithium carbonate therapy. N Engl J Med 287:867–869, 1972

Tseng HL: Interstitial myocarditis probably related to lithium carbonate intoxication. Archives of Pathology 92:444–448, 1971

Van de Merwe TJ, Silverstone T, Ankier SI, et al: A double-blind noncrossover placebo-controlled study between group comparison of trazodone and amitriptyline on cardiovascular function in major depressive disorder. Psychopathology 17(Suppl 2):64–76, 1984

Wellens H, Cats V, Duren D: Symptomatic sinus mode abnormalities following lithium carbonate therapy. Am J Med 59:285–287, 1975

White K, O'Leary J, Razani J, et al: Electrocardiographic effects of tranylcypromine versus amitriptyline. J Clin Psychiatry 44:91–93, 1983

Wilson J, Krau E, Bailas M, et al: Reversible sinus node abnormalities due to lithium carbonate therapy. N Engl J Med 294:1223–1224, 1976

Zavodnick S: Atrial flutter with amoxapine: a case report. Am J Psychiatry 138:1503–1504, 1981

Chapter 6

Mood Disorders in Post-Stroke Patients

Robert G. Robinson, M.D.
John R. Lipsey, M.D.
Thomas R. Price, M.D.

Chapter 6

Mood Disorders in Post-Stroke Patients

For many years clinicians have recognized that depressive disorders can accompany brain injury such as stroke. Bleuler (1951) and Kraepelin (1915) described the severe and long-lasting nature of these disorders. Epidemiological studies by Kay (1962) showed that there was a frequent association between stroke and first episodes of severe depression in the elderly, and Post (1962) reported, in a study of depressed geriatric patients, that many of these mood disorders followed a stroke. In spite of this recognition that depression can accompany cerebrovascular injury to the brain, there have been few systematic studies of the symptoms, course, and treatment of these depressive disorders. In addition, there has been a general assumption that these depressive disorders represent an understandable reaction to the loss or impairment of function (Benson and Geschwind 1975; Heilman 1964) rather than a neurophysiological response of the injured brain. Over the past several years we have been systematically studying these disorders and attempting to identify effective treatments as well as possible mechanisms.

CLINICAL SIGNIFICANCE

If post-stroke depressions are to be clinically significant, they must be severe, occur in a significant number of patients, and last for prolonged periods of time. That is, transient depressions that last only a few days or mild depressions that occur in a small minority of stroke patients would be much less important to clinicians than

This work has been supported in part by Research Scientist Development Awards (RGR) MH00163, NS15178, NS18862, NS16332, and MH15330 from the National Institute of Mental Health.

We thank Curtis Smith for help with the statistics and Paula Bolduc for typing the manuscript.

severe, long-lasting depressions occurring in a great number of stroke patients.

We have addressed the issue of duration of depression in two separate studies. In a follow-up study of 103 outpatients attending a stroke clinic, we found that two-thirds of the patients who were depressed at the time of the initial evaluation remained depressed for eight to nine months (Robinson and Price 1982). By one year after the initial evaluation, none of the originally depressed patients remained so. This work suggested that there was a long-standing depression which occurred in some stroke patients and that the depression had a natural course, with spontaneous remission generally occurring within one year. The second study was a prospective study of 103 acute stroke patients, in which we found that 95 percent of the patients who were depressed during the acute hospitalization remained significantly depressed at six-months' follow up (Robinson et al. 1984a). This study confirmed our earlier finding that post-stroke depressive disorders are long-lasting.

We have found two important variables which are related to the prevalence of post-stroke depression. The first is the location of the brain injury, and the second is the amount of time since the stroke. Although patients with any lesion location can have severe depressions, we have found that patients with left-frontal brain injury are the most likely to develop severe depression (Robinson et al. 1984b). During the acute stroke period, approximately 60 percent of patients with left-frontal brain injury had clinically significant depressions, as determined by meeting *Diagnostic and Statistical Manual of Mental Disorders* (DSM-III) (American Psychiatric Association 1980) diagnostic symptom criteria for major depression. In addition, among the patients with left-frontal brain injury, computerized tomography scan analysis has shown that the closer the lesion is to the frontal pole, the more severe the depression (Robinson et al. 1984b). This finding that depression severity tends to be greater as the stroke is closer to the left-frontal pole has held up even when we examined patients with traumatic (Robinson and Szetela 1981) or bilateral brain injury (Lipsey et al. 1983). In contrast, during the acute stroke period, only about 15 percent of right-hemisphere brain-injured patients have significant depressive symptoms (Robinson et al. 1984b). Thus, we have found that both *inter-* and *intra*hemisphere lesion locations were important in determining the prevalence of post-stroke depression.

We have assessed the severity of depression in two ways. The first was to compare the symptoms of post-stroke depression to the clinical symptoms used in the diagnostic criteria for major or dysthymic (minor) depression in DSM-III (American Psychiatric Association 1980). Secondly, we have quantified the depression using the various depression rating scales. If a significant depressive disorder is defined as one that meets the diagnostic criteria for either major or minor depression, we found that during the acute hospitalization, 26 percent of 103 consecutively admitted stroke patients had the symptoms of major depression, while 20 percent had the symptoms of minor (dysthymic) depression (Robinson et al. 1983b). Using depression rating scales, scores varied from no significant depression to severe depression. Thus, both the clinical diagnostic criteria and the depression rating scales indicate that almost half of acute stroke patients have clinically diagnosable depression, and about one-quarter have a severe form of depression.

The other variable which has affected the prevalence of post-stroke depression is the amount of time since the stroke. In the outpatient follow-up study described previously (Robinson and Price 1982), we found that patients between six months and two years post-stroke had a significantly increased prevalence of depression. During this time period, 45 percent of patients were depressed. In addition, from our prospective study of acute stroke patients, we found that during the first six months post-stroke, the prevalence of major or minor depression increased from 47 to 60 percent (Robinson et al. 1984a). Thus, the period of high risk for developing post-stroke depression extends over the first two years post-stroke.

DIAGNOSIS

Post-stroke depression is not often recognized in patients and even less often treated (Feibel and Springer 1982). The reasons for this may include the fact that sometimes patients do not bring up their complaints, believing as their doctors do that these feelings are all part of the disease. Other patients have multiple somatic complaints, all of which may be appropriate to the stroke deficit, leaving little time to the practitioner to ask questions about depressions.

The diagnosis of post-stroke depression, like the diagnosis of depression in patients without brain injury, is based on the existence of a cluster of symptoms which define the disorder. We have, in our research studies, divided patients into those with major depressive symptoms and those with minor depressive symptoms (Robinson et al. 1983a). The reason that we have separated them into major and minor depressions is that they appear to have different mechanisms or at least different associated variables. For instance, minor depressions are associated with posterior lesions of either the right or left hemisphere, while major depressions are strongly associated with left-frontal brain injury (Robinson et al. 1984b). In addition, major but not minor depression appears to produce a "pseudo-dementia" in stroke patients (Robinson et al. in press).

We have recently examined the utility of the dexamethasone suppression test (DST) in the evaluation of post-stroke depression (Lipsey et al. in press). Sixty-five patients with acute and chronic stroke were examined. Sixty-seven percent of the patients with symptoms of major depression who were less than one year post-stroke failed to suppress serum cortisol following dexamethasone administration. Only 25 percent of the patients with minor depression and 32 percent of the nondepressed patients failed to suppress cortisol. This finding again emphasizes the need for distinguishing major from minor post-stroke depression. The sensitivity of the DST for major depression was 67 percent but the specificity was only 70 percent. False-positive tests seemed to be related to large lesion volumes. Thus, the DST does not appear to be useful diagnostically but may provide a research tool for examining more homogeneous groups of depressed patients.

Table 1 shows the percentage of patients with a diagnosis of either major or minor depression who showed these symptoms. All patients, of course, had the symptom of sadness or depression. The next most frequent symptoms in patients with major depression were diurnal mood variation, loss of energy, anxiety, weight loss, and early morning awakening. Other prominent symptoms in patients with major depression included social withdrawal, irritability, and feelings of hopelessness. Patients with minor depressive disorders also showed symptoms of depression. However, in addition to depression, these patients had anxiety symptoms and worrying, and a smaller percentage had vegetative symptoms of sleep or appetite disturbance or decrease in libido.

In summary, the diagnosis of post-stroke depression should be made based on the existence of a cluster of symptoms. The fact that some depressions may be more severe than others should be recognized, and our data would suggest that differentiating patients into either major or minor depressive symptom categories may be useful.

ETIOLOGY

The etiology of post-stroke depressions remains undetermined. Our studies have suggested several variables which are associated with post-stroke depression; however, whether these factors are etiologically significant or whether they are merely associated findings has not been demonstrated. Probably the most fundamental question

Table 1. Distribution of Symptoms in Patients with Major or Minor Depressions

Major Depression (N = 41)	Percentage with Symptom	Minor Depression (N = 40)	Percentage with Symptom
Depressed mood	100	Depressed mood	100
Diurnal mood variation	76	Anxious, restless, worried	67
Loss of energy	73	Diurnal mood variation	46
Anxious, restless, worried	73	Hopelessness	46
Weight loss, decreased appetite	63	Loss of energy	43
Early morning awakening	56	Delayed sleep onset	33
Delayed sleep onset	56	Early morning awakening	26
Social withdrawal	54	Social withdrawal	23
Irritability	54	Weight loss, decreased appetite	15
Hopelessness	49	Self-depreciation	13
Inefficient thinking	49	Suicidal thoughts	8

about the etiology of post-stroke depressions is whether they represent an understandable psychological response to the impairment, or whether they represent a physiological reaction of the brain to focal injury. In addition to this biological or nonbiological question, there are other questions which must be investigated in determining the etiology of these disorders. For instance, what implications does the dynamic nature of post-stroke depressions have for the etiology of these disorders? That is, post-stroke depression increases in its prevalence over the first six months post-stroke, and it is uncertain whether the etiology may be different during the acute stroke period as opposed to the more chronic post-stroke period. Another issue is whether there are several etiologies to post-stroke depression. That is, depression associated with left-hemisphere brain injury may have a different etiology than depression associated with a right-hemisphere infarct. Another possibility in the etiology of post-stroke depressions is that they may be multifactorial. In other words, depression may be the outcome of various additive factors.

At this point, we can say that there appear to be several factors which influence the occurrence and severity of post-stroke depression. These include lesion location, time since stroke, severity of intellectual impairment, severity of functional physical impairment, the quality of the social supports available to the patient, and the patient's age (Robinson et al. 1984b; Robinson et al 1983b). However, although all of these variables seem to be associated with depression, there are several lines of evidence which suggest that in some post-stroke depressions the severity of impairment is not a sufficient explanation for the etiology of the depression. These lines of evidence include the fact that lesion location, both interhemispheric and intrahemispheric, is the single factor which correlates most highly with the presence and severity of depression. Secondly, although virtually all stroke lesions are associated with some level of physical or cognitive impairment, there is no single physical or cognitive impairment which is exclusively associated with depression. That is, although some patients with left-frontal brain injury have Broca's aphasia, not all of them do (Robinson et al. 1984b; Robinson and Benson 1981); although some patients with severe functional physical or cognitive impairments are depressed, not all of them are. Thus, it is most likely that biological, psychological, and social factors all contribute to post-stroke depression. Some factors are probably more important in some patients' depressions that others and it will require further work to determine the most important variables in different patients.

As one possible explanation for the etiology of post-stroke depressions, we have hypothesized that the focal brain injury may cause partial damage to the catecholamine-containing neurons in the brain, thus causing the entire catecholamine system in the brain to temporarily shut down (Robinson and Coyle 1980). Since there is a large amount of data that has implicated catecholamines in depressive disorders, this hypothesis is consistent with what we know about the biological mechanisms involved in severe functional depressions. We have also demonstrated from laboratory work that stroke injury in the rat will produce widespread changes in catecholamines throughout the brain, supporting the possibility that neurochemical changes occurring within the brain may contribute to the etiology of some post-stroke depressions (Robinson and Coyle 1980).

TREATMENT

Although post-stroke depressive disorders can be quite severe in their symptoms and last for prolonged periods of time, many of these patients do not receive treatment. The work of Feibel and Springer (1982) as well as our own studies have indicated that, in the usual course of medical care of stroke patients, most of the depressed patients do not receive treatment.

Anecdotal reports have indicated that both tricyclic antidepressants and stimulant medications (Ross and Rush 1981; Finkelstein et al. 1982) may be useful in the treatment of these disorders, as well as the use of group-therapy techniques (Oradei and Waite 1974).

We have recently reported a successful double-blind treatment study of post-stroke depression using the tricyclic antidepressant nortriptyline (Lipsey et al. 1984). In this study, half of the 34 patients had major depression. Depression was measured by the Hamilton Depression Rating scale, Zung Depression scale, Present State Examination, and an overall depression scale. Over the course of a six-week treatment period, patients treated with nortriptyline (a single oral dose, between 20 and 100 mg, given daily just before sleep) showed significantly greater improvement in depression than a similar group of patients treated with placebo. Differences between active and placebo treatment were not evident until more than two weeks after therapy began. Patients treated with nortriptyline had serum drug levels between 50 and 140 ng/ml (the therapeutic range for function depressions) at four and six weeks after starting treatment. In three patients on active medication, delirium with drowsiness, confusion, and sometimes agitation developed. All these symptoms, however, cleared within days after discontinuing nortriptyline. Contraindications to treatment included severe cardiac arrhythmias, recent myocardial infarction, heart block, urinary outlet obstruction, and narrow angle glaucoma. The findings indicate, however, that treatment of post-stroke depression with nortriptyline, if done with care, can be a significant addition to the treatments available to stroke patients.

SUMMARY

Post-stroke depression is common, often severe, and long-lasting. It can often go unrecognized if patients' moods are not specifically examined. Post-stroke depression can be diagnosed by asking the patient about the symptoms of depression, and these depressions have now been shown to be treatable with nortriptyline. Although the etiology has not been determined, the association between depression and lesion location is much stronger than the association with severity of physical or intellectual impairment. Left-frontal lesions are strongly related to depression and the closer the lesion is to the frontal pole the more severe the depression.

REFERENCES

American Psychiatric Association: Diagnostic and Statistical Manual of Mental Disorders, 3rd ed. Washington, DC, American Psychiatric Association, 1980

Benson DF, Geschwind N: Psychiatric conditions associated with focal lesions of the central nervous system, in The American Handbook of Psychiatry, Vol 4. Edited by Reiser MF. New York, Basic Books, 1975, pp 208–243

Bleuler EP: Textbook of Psychiatry. New York, Dover, 1951, pp 230–242, 343–344

Feibel JH and Springer CJ: Depression and failure to resume social activities after stroke. Arch Phys Med Rehabil 63:276–277, 1982

Finkelstein S, Benowitz LI, Baldessarini R, et al: Mood, vegetative disturbance, and dexamethasone suppression test after stroke. Ann Neurol 12:463–468, 1982

Heilman KM: Neuropsychologic changes in the stroke patient. Geriatrics 29:153–160, 1964

Kay DWK: Outcome and cause of death in mental disorders of old age: a long-term follow-up of functional and organic psychoses. Acta Psychiatr Scand 38:249–267, 1962

Kraepelin E: Clinical Psychiatry. New York, Macmillan, 1915, pp 335–336, 343–344

Lipsey JR, Robinson RG, Pearlson GD, et al: Mood change following bilateral hemisphere brain injury. Br J Psychiatry 143:266–273, 1983

Lipsey JR, Robinson RG, Pearlson GD, et al: Nortriptyline treatment of post-stroke depression: a double-blind study. Lancet 1:297–300, 1984

Lipsey JR, Robinson RG, Pearlson GD, et al: Dexamethasone suppression test and mood following stroke. Am J Psychiatry (in press)

Oradei DM, Waite NS: Group psychotherapy with stroke patients during the immediate recovery phase. Am J Orthopsychiatry 44:386–395, 1974

Post R: The significance of affective symptoms in old age, Maudsley Monograph, No. 10. London, Oxford University Press, 1962

Robinson RG, Benson DF: Depression in aphasic patients: frequency, severity, and clinical–pathological correlations. Brain Lang 14:282–291, 1981

Robinson RG, Coyle JT: The differential effect of right versus left hemispheric cerebral infarction on catecholamines and behavior in the rat. Brain Res 188:63–78, 1980

Robinson RG, Price TR: Post-stroke depressive disorders: a follow-up study of 103 patients. Stroke 13:635–641, 1982

Robinson RG, Szetela B: Mood change following left hemisphere brain injury. Ann Neurol 9:447–453, 1981

Robinson RG, Kubos KL, Starr LB, et al: Mood changes in stroke patients: relationship to lesion location. Compr Psychiatry 24:555–556, 1983a

Robinson RG, Starr LB, Kubos KL, et al: A two-year longitudinal study of post-stroke mood disorders: findings during the initial evaluation. Stroke 14:736–744, 1983b

Robinson RG, Starr LB, Price TR: A two-year longitudinal study of post-stroke mood disorders: prevalence and duration at six months follow-up. Br J Psychiatry 144:256–262, 1984a

Robinson RG, Kubos KL, Starr LB, et al: Mood disorders in stroke patients. Brain 107:81–93, 1984b

Robinson RG, Bolla-Wilson K, Kaplan E, et al: Evidence for intellectual impairment related to depression in stroke patients. Br J Psychiatry (in press)

Ross ED, Rush AJ: Diagnosis and neuroanatomical correlates of depression in brain damaged patients. Arch Gen Psychiatry 38:1344–1354, 1981

Chapter 7

Kidney and Lithium Therapy in the Elderly

Abdol H. Samiy, M.D.

Chapter 7

Kidney and Lithium Therapy in the Elderly

The use of lithium in the treatment of affective disorders in the elderly is generally well accepted. However, there are limited data in the literature dealing with indications, contraindications, and side effects of lithium therapy in the elderly. The range of toxicity of lithium therapy in the elderly is essentially the same as in younger patients. But, in view of probable difference in lithium disposition and significant age-induced pathophysiological alterations in the elderly, it is likely that elderly patients treated with lithium may be subject to a number of special problems and hazards.

This chapter will focus specifically on renal problems associated with lithium therapy. It will describe age-induced changes in kidney function, renal effects of chronic lithium therapy, body disposition of lithium, and finally, renal evaluation and monitoring of patients before and after treatment with lithium.

AGE-INDUCED ALTERATION IN KIDNEY FUNCTION

Animal studies have shown that aging is accompanied by significant structural alterations of the kidneys—characterized by focal or segmental glomerulosclerosis, an increase in mesangial matrix, thickening of glomerular basement membrane (GBM), and epithelial cell foot-process fusion (Berg 1965). In addition, renal tubules demonstrate increased thickness of the basement membrane and dilatation (Ashworth et al. 1960; Coleman and Barthold 1972). In humans, age-induced structural changes in the kidneys consist of progressive loss of renal mass, mainly in the cortical region of the kidneys (Rowe 1980). The number of glomeruli falls and the volume of mesangium gradually increases with advancing age (Sorenson 1977; Tauchi 1971). There is also an increase in thickness of GBM and tubular basement membrane. Considerable sclerotic changes in renal vasculature have been reported with aging even in the absence of hypertension or other systemic diseases (Daramady 1973).

Accompanying these structural changes, there is a gradual decline in renal function (Everitt 1958; Friedman 1972; Solomon 1973). After age 40, there is a gradual decline in kidney function manifested by a fall in plasma flow (RPF), and in glomerular filtration rate (GFR), and in renal reabsorptive capacity (Rowe 1980). Similarly, there is a decrease in normal renal–endocrine functions. It should be noted that these functional alterations are not accompanied by any significant symptoms or signs. However, aging kidneys have a reduced capacity to adapt to rapid hemodynamic changes resulting from diseases particularly when associated with disturbances in water and electrolytes.

RENAL HANDLING OF LITHIUM

An important consequence of deterioration in renal function is altered handling of a large number of drugs and their active or inactive metabolites. This is particularly important in consideration of lithium, which is excreted almost entirely by the kidneys. After filtration lithium is reabsorbed in the proximal tubules (Thomsen and Schou 1968). Since furosemide, a loop diuretic, increases the fractional excretion of lithium, it is inferred that lithium is probably reabsorbed by the loop of Henle. Factors which alter tubular reabsorption of lithium will affect serum lithium levels. For instance, diuretics, such as chlorothiazide, which change reabsorption of salt in the proximal tubules, will modify tubular reabsorption of lithium and affect the serum level of lithium.

It is evident that age-induced alteration in renal function has an important impact on lithium disposition and consequently on treatment of elderly patients with lithium. The effect of age on lithium therapy has been the subject of several studies. In one study 82 psychiatric outpatients with an age range of 21 to 84 were investigated during lithium therapy (Hewick 1977). In patients older than 50 years, daily lithium dose required to give a similar plasma level was significantly lower than in patients of a younger age group. In patients aged 70 to 79 years, the required dose was 31 percent lower than in patients younger than 50. In this study, a 50 percent reduction in lithium dosage was necessary to reduce the high incidence of side effects and to maintain lithium in the lower therapeutic range. In another work, the plasma clearance and volume of distribution of lithium was studied in six elderly patients on chronic lithium therapy (Chapron 1982). This study revealed a significant decrease in renal plasma clearance of lithium, probably as a result of age-induced renal function changes, and a reduction in volume of distribution of lithium as a consequence of a decrease in muscle mass of the elderly. These alterations considerably prolong the half-life of lithium. A 50 percent dosage reduction appears to be appropriate to compensate for an age-related decrease in lithium excretion and to reduce serious adverse effects of lithium.

RENAL EFFECTS OF LITHIUM

The effects of lithium treatment on kidneys have been extensively studied in patients of all age groups, but most of the studies have been carried out in younger patients. The structural and functional renal alterations with lithium are probably similar in younger and older age groups. It is likely, however, that age-related renal changes and significantly different lithium pharmacokinetics will adversely affect the severity of nephrotoxicity of lithium in elderly patients.

It is generally accepted that chronic lithium therapy results in significant histological changes in the kidneys. However, there is very little evidence that these changes are persistent or progressive. No case of chronic renal failure has been reported so far with chronic use of lithium. Structural changes reported with lithium therapy consist of ballooning vacuolation of the cytoplasm with pyknotic nuclei. Tubular cells show desquamation of distal tubules. Focal nephron atrophy, sclerosis of glomeruli, and interstitial fibrosis have been reported by several investigators (Hestbech et al. 1977; Burrows et al. 1978; Lindop and Padfield 1975).

These structural changes of lithium therapy are associated with significant renal dysfunction, which may be manifested clinically in various forms. First, patients on short-term lithium therapy often develop polyuria. Polyuria can result from lithium-induced naturesis and inhibition of aldosterone. But the most common cause of polyuria is antidiuretic-hormone (ADH)-resistant or nephrogenic diabetes insipidus. The serum level of ADH in these patients is normal or even elevated. Patients with nephrogenic diabetes insipidus have a considerable polydypsia and a marked polyuria—usually in the range of three to six liters per 24 hours. Glomerular filtration rate (GFR) remains normal. Polyuria is usually reversible and will improve with discontinuation of lithium therapy (Angrist et al. 1970; Lee et al. 1971; Price and Beisswenger 1978).

Nephrotic syndrome has also been reported in a few patients on chronic lithium therapy (Moskovitz 1981). In these cases, renal biopsy showed pathological alterations of minimal-change disease. Nephrotic syndrome and proteinuria disappear when lithium is discontinued (Richmond et al. 1980).

A more serious adverse effect of chronic lithium therapy is permanent renal damage with irreversible deterioration of renal function. In one study, 14 patients on recurrent lithium therapy for a two- to 14-year period were investigated (Hestbech et al. 1977). Thirteen of these patients showed focal nephron atrophy, glomerulosclerosis, and interstitial fibrosis when compared to age-matched controls. In another study, it was shown that 32 out of 110 patients who received lithium for six months or longer had polyuria and a fall in GFR (Hansen and Amdisen 1978). Similar findings were reported in other studies (Burrows et al. 1978).

There are, however, a number of unsettled problems regarding the study of long-term effects of lithium on the kidneys. First, in most of these studies there was no proper control of age-matched psychiatric patients. Furthermore, it has been shown that patients with serious psychiatric illness may be at a greater risk of developing renal disease (Kincaid-Smith 1979). Second, a large number of psychiatric patients, including those on chronic lithium treatment, may be taking other drugs, including psychotropic agents, with possible nephrotoxic effects. Third, histological changes reported in kidneys of lithium-treated patients are nonspecific and not unlike those seen with analgesic nephropathy. Finally, many studies do not exclude the existence of renal disease before lithium therapy was initiated.

The toxicity of lithium therapy in older patients appears to be generally greater and more frequent than in younger patients. In one study of hospitalized elderly patients, moderate to severe side effects were reported even when serum lithium level was within or minimally higher than the therapeutic range (Roose et al. 1979). Neurotoxicity was the most common complication in this age group. The effect of chronic lithium therapy on renal function of the elderly patient has not been adequately studied. Hospital charts of 62 patients receiving long-term lithium therapy were reviewed by an investigator studying the effect of lithium on renal function (Hai-Gwo et al. 1980). They reported that there was a tendency for older patients to show a greater increase in serum creatinine at follow-up than the normal control. In our own study of 20 patients treated with chronic lithium therapy, all of the five elderly patients included showed a significant fall in creatinine clearance in contrast to only a few younger patients (Samiy and Brown, manuscript submitted for publication).

It can be postulated that the higher incidence of primary kidney disease and systemic disorders with renal involvement in the elderly, the existence of age-induced renal dysfunction, and multiple drug therapy may render these elderly patients more vulnerable to development of renal damage with chronic lithium therapy.

Interaction between lithium and diuretics has been already mentioned. With frequent use of diuretics in elderly patients the importance of interaction between these two drugs should be further emphasized.

Since lithium is mainly reabsorbed by the proximal renal tubules, the interaction between lithium and diuretics is based on the effect of the latter on tubular reabsorption of the former. There are several classes of diuretics, each with a different rate of action in the renal tubules. Furosemide, a loop diuretic that increases sodium excretion in the proximal tubules, results in a decreased lithium reabsorption and enhanced lithium excretion. In contrast, chlorothiazide, which increases sodium excretion in the distal tubules, brings about a compensatory increase in proximal sodium reabsorption—and a parallel increase in lithium reabsorption. In patients being treated with diuretics such as chlorothiazide, the use of lithium should be initiated and maintained with caution. The dosage of lithium may need to be adjusted, with frequent monitoring of serum lithium level.

KIDNEY FUNCTION EVALUATION AND MONITORING

Thus it is essential that before lithium therapy is initiated, renal function should be carefully evaluated in patients of all age groups—but particularly in the elderly. The most common laboratory test currently employed for measuring renal function is serum creatinine level. It is important to be aware that with increasing age there is a decrease in muscle mass and consequently a fall in serum creatinine level. Therefore, age-induced decline in renal function may not be reflected in an increase in serum creatinine.

Determination of serum creatinine is not an accurate marker of renal glomerular function in general and in the elderly patients in particular. Creatinine clearance is a more sensitive test but it is technically more difficult to perform because of the need for an accurate 24-hour urine collection. It was recently shown that determination of serum B_2-microglobulin level may be a more sensitive guide to renal glomerular function (Carrie et al. 1980). We recently demonstrated that serum B_2-microglobulin level more accurately reflects alterations in GFR in patients on chronic lithium therapy (Samiy and Brown in press).

Poor renal function, as indicated by an elevated serum creatinine and B_2-microglobulin or a low creatinine clearance, is considered a relative contraindication to lithium therapy for two important reasons. First, when treated with lithium, patients with poor renal function have a greater risk of developing various adverse effects. Second, there is the possibility of a greater incidence of nephropathy in patients who already have some degree of renal dysfunction.

In the elderly there is a greater incidence of primary renal disease and of systemic diseases with renal involvement. The presence of these disorders may further affect the renal functions resulting in a greater decrease in renal clearance of lithium. Similarly, diuretics, nonsteroidal anti-inflammatory drugs, and a number of other medications taken by elderly patients may reduce renal clearance of lithium and increase the serum lithium level. With an increase in serum lithium, not only is there a greater incidence of lithium toxicity but also an increased serum lithium level, which may result in additional renal damage. Furthermore many elderly patients are placed on a salt-restricted diet. The renal reabsorption of lithium increases in these patients and results in a higher serum lithium level and a greater risk of developing lithium toxicity.

In view of the insensitivity of serum creatinine, and despite difficulty in 24-hour urine collection, it is advisable to obtain a baseline creatinine clearance and a serum B_2-microglobulin in the elderly patients. Periodic assessment of renal function at intervals of three to six months is essential. Occasionally an increase in serum lithium level may indicate an early decline in renal function and may actually precede a change in serum creatinine.

In conclusion, lithium is a widely accepted drug for treatment of affective disorders in the elderly. With age-induced pathophysiological alterations in the elderly, there is a great incidence of toxicity, particularly neurotoxicity, even when the serum level of lithium is maintained at essentially normal range. With advancing age, not only is there a gradual decline in renal function, but increasing incidence of systemic diseases; thus there is a greater risk of secondary kidney disease and dysfunction. Elderly patients often receive multiple drugs, such as diuretics, which may have considerable effects on renal excretion of lithium and on the kidney functions. All these factors combine to increase the risk of nephrotoxicity in the elderly patient. The renal function of elderly patients should be initially evaluated and periodically monitored during the course of therapy. Despite many hazards, lithium can be used safely in elderly patients if there is an understanding of lithium pharmacokinetics and an appreciation for potential renal toxicity of lithium.

REFERENCES

Angrist, BM, Gershon S, Levitan SJ, et al: Lithium-induced diabetes insipidus-like syndrome. Compr Psychiatry 11:141–146, 1970

Ashworth CT, Erdmann RR, Arnold BS: Age changes in the renal basement membrane in rats. Am J Pathol 36:165–171, 1960

Berg BN: Spontaneous nephrosis with proteinuria, hyperglobinemia, hypercholesteremia in the rat. Proc Soc Exp Biol Med 119:417–427, 1965

Burrows GD, Davies B, Kincaid-Smith P: Unique tubular lesions after lithium. Lancet 1:1310C, 1978

Carrie JB, Golbetz HV, Michaels AS, et al: Creatinine: an inadequate filtration marker in glomerular disease. Am J Med 69:177–182, 1980

Chapron DJ, Cameron IR, White LB: Observation on lithium disposition in the elderly. J Am Geriatr Soc 30:651–655, 1982

Coleman GL, Barthold SW, Osbaldiston GW, et al: Pathological changes during aging in barrier-reared Fisher 344 male rats. Gerontology 32:258–278, 1977

Daramady EM, Offer J, Woodhouse MA: The parameters of the aging kidneys. J Pathol 109:195–207, 1973

Everitt AV: The urinary excretion of protein, nonprotein nitrogen, creatinine and uric acid in aging male rats. Gerontology 2:33–46, 1958

Friedman SA, Raizner AE, Solomon N: Functional defects in aging kidney. Ann Intern Med 76:41–45, 1972

Hai-GWO HWU, Ardekani AB, Helzer JE: A longitudinal record study of renal function in patients treated with lithium. J Affective Disord 3:101–109, 1981

Hansen HE, Amdisen A: Lithium intoxication: report of 23 cases and review of 100 cases from the literature. Q J Med 186:123–144, 1978

Hestbech H, Hansen HE, Amdisen A, et al: Chronic renal lesions following long-term treatment with lithium. Kidney Int 12:205–213, 1977

Hewick DS, Newbury P, Hopewood S, et al: Age as a factor affecting lithium therapy. Br J Clin Pharmacol 4:201–205, 1977

Kincaid-Smith P: Renal biopsy in lithium and pre-lithium patients. Lancet 2:700–701, 1979

Lee RV, Jampol LM, Brown WN: Nephrogenic diabetes insipidus in lithium intoxication: complication of lithium therapy. N Engl J Med 284:93–94, 1971

Lindop GBH, Padfield PL: The renal pathology in a case of lithium-induced diabetes insipidus. J Clin Pathol 28:472–475, 1975

Moskovitz R: Lithium-induced nephrotic syndrome. Am J Psychiatry 183:382–383, 1981

Price TA, Beisswenger PJ: Lithium and diabetes insipidus. Ann Intern Med 88:576–577, 1978

Richmond AV, Masco HL, Rifkin SI: Minimal-change disease in the nephrotic syndrome associated with lithium therapy. Ann Intern Med 92:70–72, 1980

Roose SP, Bone S. Haidorfer C, et al: Lithium treatment in older patients. Am J Psychiatry 36:843–844, 1979

Rowe JW: Aging and renal function. Annual Review of Gerontology and Geriatrics 1:161–179, 1980

Solomon P: The effects of age in reducing renal functions. Geriatrics 28:83-87, 1973

Sorenson F: Quantitative studies of the renal corpuscle. Acta Pathol Microbiol Scand (A) 585:356–366, 1977

Tauchi H, Tsuboik, Okutomi J: Age changes in the human kidney of different races. Gerontology 17:87–97, 1971

Thomsen K, Schou M: Renal lithium excretion in man. Am J Physiol 215:823–827, 1968